Complexity in Healthcare and the Language of Consultation

Exploring the other side of medicine

Derek Steinberg

Formerly, Consultant Child and Adolescent Psychiatrist, The Bethlem Royal and Maudsley Hospitals, London

Radcliffe Publishing
Oxford • Seattle

Radcliffe Publishing Ltd
18 Marcham Road
Abingdon
Oxon OX14 1AA
United Kingdom

www.radcliffe-oxford.com
Electronic catalogue and worldwide online ordering facility.

British Library Cataloguing in Publication Data

A catalogue record for this book is available from the British Library.

ISBN 1 85775 854 4

Typeset by Acorn Bookwork Ltd, Salisbury, Wiltshire
Printed and bound by TJ International Ltd, Padstow, Cornwall

Contents

The Secret of Success is the Organisation of the Non-Obvious

Chinese motto in a Christmas cracker

The Map is not the Territory

Jean Baudrillard

Preface and acknowledgements

First, the quotes on the previous page. I found the first in a Christmas cracker at a time when I was trying to make sense of working in child and adolescent psychiatry. In a busy service with a long waiting list (it doesn't matter which one because at the time they were mostly rather similar) children waited for months for an appointment which took up much of a morning or afternoon, at the end of which they might be told (pretty accurately) that there was nothing much wrong, or that the problem was primarily in the family or the school – or had been, because things might have got worse, and then better, during the wait. By then, whether there was a diagnosis of serious disorder or no disorder at all, indeed sometimes by the time of the first referral letter, the boy or girl would have accumulated previous helpers: social workers, community physicians, community nurses, probation officers, psychotherapists and counsellors, health visitors, paediatricians, previous child psychiatrists, remedial teachers and occasionally lawyers, some of these experts more appropriately than others, some more helpful than others, and several coming or going because of the kinds of change that happen in health and care services – a consultant hands the child over to a colleague, who then 'rotates' elsewhere; a social worker is just about to leave and hands over to a colleague, who then finds that he or she isn't in the right team for the child's 'needs'; or the address is wrong, the child changes class, or the teacher changes class.

The model of care was the kaleidoscope; indeed, a kind of double kaleidoscope, because just as a whole range of different things in terms of the assessment could be said about each child and family (from nothing wrong to everything wrong, and in terms of development, or individual psychology, or illness, or family or school relationships), what was available was similarly in some kind of orbit. So a child enmeshed in a dysfunctional family might be seen by a psychologist whose preferred approach is behavioural; or a boy or girl with a habit problem or a disorder of brain biochemistry might be seen by a family therapy team. Or the team most willing and able to help might turn out to be in the wrong catchment area, or someone else in the multidisciplinary team might have second thoughts about whether they were really 'right' for the child; or they too had a key member leaving; or the child's birth date would only be all right for that unit for another week. Or the child or family couldn't get on with X; or vice versa. I once wrote a small book about it which some people said was all right, and others said was all wrong.

Now here's the first point: nearly all the people I can think of were conscientious, competent, well-meaning people doing their best; but the treatment systems didn't match the range and kinds of problem and the complexity of their nature, being based as much in several people's attitudes, knowledge and beliefs as in very different contributions by biological, psychodynamic, cognitive, family, educational and *service* variables – particularly the latter. On the subject of child psychiatry, one should mention the enormously important introduction of the multi-axial diagnostic system, each axis representing psychiatric, intellectual, developmental, physical disorder and social factors; but the *values* attached to each and the way different clinical teams preferred to respond tended to leave a gap between what the clinic wanted to do and the complexity of the child's and family's case. Whatever was wrong, or not wrong, in the child seemed ill-met and sometimes amplified by the way care and treatment was organised – and I mean organised in our thinking rather than organised on paper. I introduced the idea of putting alongside our well tried and tested diagnostic systems (pretty good, in child psychiatry, and properly multifactorial) a simpler system of my own: Who is concerned about what? And why? And who is in a position to help? It was problem-oriented, in plain English, and the answers did not replace the clinical assessment but ran alongside it (Steinberg 1983, 1987, 2000c; Tyrer and Steinberg, 2005). It was about organising the fuller, fuzzier picture, that which was not at first obvious, and it led to my interest in a systems approach, which just seemed properly matched to psychological, socio-cultural and biological systems, in themselves and in their interaction.

The second point is that my own general medical experience plus various perspectives of it as doctor, relative and friend of patients, and occasional patient myself, is that what was amplified by child, adolescent and family psychiatry's particularly acute and upfront crises, its legal and ethical dilemmas, the many uncertainties and the unknowable in child care and therapy, and the many people (family and professionals) involved, seemed to throw a bit of light on problems in other medical and health fields too. In fact, child psychiatry does a pretty good job in trying to make sense of the contemporary complexity and chaos of child upbringing, behaviour, health and all the opinions, misinformation, problems and disasters involved. The very success of child psychiatry's boldly pioneering approach (multi-axial, multidisciplinary, multi-agency, straddling everything from biochemistry to subculture, consultative as well as clinical) to its own clientele provides some indicators, I believe, about what is on the way in the rest of medicine and healthcare. What the adult world insists children need today they will want for themselves tomorrow.

And so to the assertion by the postmodern philosopher, Jean Baudrillard that the map is not the territory. Like much that is good in supposed post-modern philosophy, it can sound bizarre because it tries to turn on its head things which are already upside down. One thinks of Magritte's painting of a pipe entitled 'This is Not a Pipe'. Indeed it isn't, when you think about it, and it is the surprise that makes you think about it. Thus, I don't get the impression that the appearance on paper or computer screens of railway timetables is the same subject as organising rolling stock to run along tracks and what happens on platforms; nor that piles of papers bound together into Action Plans or Initiatives or Projects for agriculture, the law or healthcare, or just about anything else, bear more than a superficial resemblance to what goes on in farms or the streets or courts of law or hospitals. In healthcare the people who know what goes on and are person-ally curious, interested and motivated to make sense of things and put them right are healthcare workers and their clientele, there in the clinic. Systems consultation is about their negotiating together who has a problem about what, and what might be the options for dealing with it. Thus it is a 'bottom up' rather than a 'top down' model, although as soon as one identi-fies the issue as such it becomes claimable as the territory of the 'real' experts, the bottomupologists and topdowniatricians, with all the potential for papers and projects and 'tsars' and government-health community feedback-feedforward focus liaison officers; and so on. However, the clinician and the client can tell a pipe from a painting of a pipe, a wait from a waiting list, and the anticipation and feel of a surgical operation from a waiting list. Systems consultation is about asking simple questions about what actually happens, as near as we can get to the territory. And where the terrain is unclear, the answers are sought not through big management or big research but by asking more questions of those who are in the frame or needed in the frame.

Now the science, art and practice of clinical work (and I would include here the best of psychotherapy and counselling) is explicitly and commend-ably down to earth. However, its very focus, indeed its need to focus, can leave out a huge penumbra of other matters that are strongly influential on the clinical presentation and the impact of therapy. These other matters are complex and belong to very different areas, for example individual psychology, the psychodynamics of relationships, systems theory and theories of organisations and institutions, and not everyone can be inter-ested in or familiar with them all. Systems consultation provides not an overarching theory of complexity but a pragmatic way of asking about different aspects and forms of complexity; it is not about tidying up what is, in healthcare, unavoidably complex, but how to find one's way through it; how to make the most of what is *necessarily* a complex, multifactorial and dynamic field, some of it observable and measurable, some of it intuit-ive. This is what this book is about: not a grand plan to make sense of all the chaos and complexity involved in healthcare, but the kind of equipment needed to navigate it, and the angle of entry into and out of it. And the idea of systems consultation presented here is as an approach *complementary* to clinical work, not as an alternative to it.

Systems consultation is a system of enquiry, not a theory; there is no unifying theoretical position. It is in a way a set of tools shaped by what it is examining; it mirrors the necessary complexities of healthcare by being multilingual, understanding the various languages of psychology, biology and social organisation and their various variations and pathologies *and* the kinds of philosophy and micro-politics that makes some sense of it all, *but* then doing its best to translate it all into plain language for the benefit of all concerned – not least its practitioners. In all these areas it has an interest in what goes on in and between clinicians and our colleagues and our clients – that emotionally heated and turbulent triad which determines what is looked at, given priority and attended to in healthcare, and is so often pushed to one side. Systems theory also takes for granted that the clinician is part of the scene, not the dispassionate, external observer of some supposedly rational thinker's fantasies. General systems theory, which informs systems consultation, corresponds with psychodynamic thinking on the one hand and quantum physics on the other in their separate discoveries that the observer is never entirely objective, being part of that which is being observed.

To this extent – the involvement of quite complex models of human functioning and behaviour – the book is complex, though I hope I am able to demonstrate something about the consultative approach by proceeding through complex and sometimes ethereal areas by posing serial and relatively straightforward questions. To the extent that there will be some repetition and going round in circles, that matches the field and the task: the explanations here are circular and reciprocal rather than linear because the problems are circular and reciprocal, rather than linear; as are relationships, and as is biology. To extend the earlier metaphor, having entered the complexity atmosphere we will have to adopt a circular route as we descend, to avoid burning up.

A particular guiding principle of my own, one that I hope justifies the complex and roundabout route of what follows, is that complexity – used properly – is the price we pay for keeping things as simple and comprehensible as we can at the clinical level. I think that if as healthcare professionals we try to 'keep things simple' by setting aside the necessary complexities of healthcare, we may get through the working day feeling that we've more or less covered the necessary ground, but the people left struggling with what's left over are our patients. It is they who carry away from the clinic a whole bagful of unanswered questions, unaddressed problems and part-solutions.

*

I would like to acknowledge my appreciation of what I have learned in training and working over the years at the Maudsley and Bethlem Royal Hospitals and in several years' training at the Tavistock Institute of Human Relations. This dual experience at two very different institutions represented for me objective attempts to make sense of mental health and disorder on the one hand, and intuitive attempts on the other; though I found more in common between them than in their much-caricatured differences. This book is an attempt to use these two sides of the brain together; this can be inconvenient academically, institutionally and conceptually, but it is the way real people work.

I am particularly indebted to the staff and participants at the early days of the Tavistock Institute's programme in consultation in community mental health (now identified as organisational consultation), and particularly for the introduction by John Bowlby and Dorothy Heard of attachment theory into our thinking and debate. Bowlby's attachment theory is, for me, the best conceptual model we have so far which straddles both psychodynamic thinking and observable social and biological behaviour. Like systems consultation, it deals with complexity by going into its roots and ramifications – not by an all-encompassing theory but by a basically straightforward basic model of understanding which shows patterns all the way from small systems to large ones. In one of these seminars Bowlby once observed that people, after first hearing him speak on these ideas, would come forward to thank him, comment that they found nothing to disagree with, but that it all sounded, bafflingly and frustratingly, 'too simple'.

I would also want to acknowledge the very many people, teachers, colleagues and students, who joined me or helped over the years in experiments in applying consultative approaches to clinical, organisational and team questions, particularly (in approximate chronological order) at the Adolescent Unit of the Maudsley and Bethlem Royal Hospital; at Adelaide House Adolescent Unit, Ladbroke Grove; for some valued teaching occasions with the Ministry of Community Development and Child Psychiatric Clinic, Singapore; with the British Council and the Ministry of Education, Trinidad and Tobago; with 'NAFSIYAT', the Intercultural Therapy Centre, London; the Arts and Therapy Centre, Athens; with the Faculty of Nursing, University of Athens; at the Departments of Child Psychiatry and Neuropsychiatry in Warsaw, Poznan and Cracow in Poland; with the Faculty of Medicine, Jiagellonian University, Cracow; with the Rowantree Foundation, particularly with the departments of Child, Adolescent and Psychiatry at Groeningen, at Breda and at Voorst in Holland; at the Kowloon Hospital and Kwai Chung Child Psychiatric Clinic, Hong Kong; and to Professor Shozo Aoki and his colleagues at the Kawasaki Medical School, Japan.

Finally, the examples given in the text in the following pages are fabricated; as I often point out in connection with systems consultation and the institutions and part-institutions it works with, it is easier to preserve the privacy and confidentiality of clients than teams and organisations, and I have done that here by a kind of collage technique, using fragments of real occasions and experiences transposed to different kinds of place. Thus, I believe, both fictional but authentic: the kinds of thing that happen.

Derek Steinberg
February 2005

About the author

As a Consultant Psychiatrist Derek Steinberg developed and led the in-patient adolescent service at the Bethlem Royal and Maudsley Hospitals, London, for 19 years before moving on to an equivalent role at The Priory Ticehurst House Hospital, Sussex, where he became Senior Clinical Tutor. His training has included experience at the Park Hospital for Children, Oxford, the National Hospitals for Neurology and Neurosurgery, and the Tavistock Institute, and for several years he was Honorary Visiting Lecturer in Psychiatry and subsequently Visiting Reader in the sociology department at the University of Surrey. This background, and his activities in the arts, reflects the view that the proper understanding of psychiatry, and of health and medicine in general, needs the broadest possible perspective, and this is reflected in the present book. He has published some 60 papers and chapters, and this is his eighth book, though some do seem to recall best his many published cartoons. He teaches nationally and internationally, particularly on the major clinical disorders of adolescence, staff training and development, and on the interrelationships between biology, psychiatry and the arts.

Other books by Derek Steinberg:

- *Using Child Psychiatry* (Hodder and Stoughton, 1981)

- *Clinical Psychiatry of Adolescence: clinical work from a social and development perspective* (John Wiley and Sons Ltd, 1983)

- *The Adolescent Unit: work and team work in adolescent psychiatry* (John Wiley and Sons Ltd, 1986)

- *Models for Mental Disorder: conceptual models in psychiatry* (with Peter Tyrer; John Wiley and Sons Ltd, 1998)

- *Basic Adolescent Psychiatry* (Blackwell, 1987)

- *Inter-Professional Consultation: innovation and imagination in working relationships* (Blackwell, 1989)

- *Letters From the Clinic: letter writing in clinical practice for mental health professionals* (Brunner–Routledge, an imprint of Taylor & Francis Group, 2000)

- *Consciousness Reconnected: missing links between neuroscience, depth psychology and the arts* (Radcliffe Publishing, forthcoming)

CHAPTER 1

Introduction: the three kinds of consultation

- Clinical, organisational and systems consultation.
- Uses of systems consultation.
- Complexities in healthcare.
- An outline of the book.

A pre-emptive summary

The 'consultation' is the focal point of clinical and therapeutic work in healthcare, but in practice and in the detail the term can mean just about anything. This book discusses three main kinds of consultation: *clinical consultation, systems or organisational consultation,* and the consultation described in the following pages and which is a kind of informed partnership between the other two.

The first, clinical consultation, is an interview designed to elicit symptoms and signs, from which the clinician can make a diagnosis and plan treatment. It is at the very least the kind of question-and-answer encounter which computer fans (largely non-clinicians) have for some years imagined was the very essence of medicine, and could be carried out more quickly and efficiently by machine, nothing getting in the way of the essential logic and objectivity of the process. It is not as simple as that, however, and doctors and others have long been preoccupied with what it takes for the clinical consultation to work, from the old (and excellent) advice to '*listen* to the patient; he is telling you the diagnosis' to accounts such as that by Pendleton *et al.* (2003). However, the core skills of clinical work are thoroughly established, central to mainstream training and already familiar as the focus of healthcare; this book is about something else.

Systems consultation has a tortuous pedigree (*see* pages 17 *et seq* and 29 *et*

1

seq). It has been known as organisational consultation, inter-professional consultation or just plain 'consultation'. This varied terminology is confusing but reflects, in the fields of health and care, developments over the years in techniques designed to help with the many extra-clinical issues that influenced diagnosis and treatment, including how we work and how we work together; the clinical interview's penumbra, as it were. As clinicians we know the importance of extending into family work; but there is another kind of family, sometimes troubled, known to be dysfunctional from time to time and often in and out of trouble with the neighbours, and that is the clinical, academic or caring team. Systems consultation was developed specifically for work with professionals and teams.

This kind of consultation can be defined as the activity undertaken when one person (the consultant) helps another (the consultee) to work more effectively, by working through the consultee's own perspective and helping to mobilise the consultee's own skills. The consultant doesn't 'take over'; it is work-focused, not personality-focused, and the consultee is not subordinate, because it is a jointly undertaken peer–peer exercise. What to do with the outcome remains a matter for the consultee. Much of the rest of this book is about exploring the implications of this working definition. Meanwhile, anyone familiar with the caution, doubts and hot and cold war-zones involved in work within and across healthcare teams and their hierarchies will see the necessity for these ground rules. They are particularly important for dealing with territorial and role issues between professionals and professional groups, and for being interested in, understanding and respecting the roles, responsibilties and perspectives of others. Not all specialists are good at this; having evolved so many highly specialised areas, which we have needed to do, we now need specialists in working across specialties.

But if systems consultation can help us as healthcare professionals to work more effectively with each other, dealing with our private doubts about it as we go, is it possible to extend this kind of curiosity, understanding and partnership to our patients and clients too? This book explores this as well. To take this question seriously needs a strategy, not intent alone, and while systems consultation would be helpful alongside the clinical approach they cannot be merged seamlessly. The special value of the systemic approach is in its fundamental distinction from the clinical perspective; its enquiries and findings are different, sufficiently so to require a different identity and role from the purely clinical one. The 'third kind of consultation' therefore is not proposed as a hybrid formed of the other two, but as a kind of binocular, two-handed approach to all healthcare issues: the well-tried, well-tested and generally well-taught clinical approach on the one hand, and the relatively new but promising systems approach on the other. So you will find in the brand new medical bag I am recommending not one new piece of equipment but a pair, and I suggest we will be needing them both in twenty-first century healthcare, whose changes, chaos, complexity and increasing difficulty is already very well under way. In medicine, and in healthcare generally, we are going to have to move very fast to catch up.

Why 'systems' consultation? The term comes from Von Bertalanffy's *General Systems Theory* (1968), which is about the homeostatic, multifactorial way living systems work. There is a brief account of its background and nature in Chapter 4.

For the moment I will describe it in these terms: when the doctor (or any other therapist) meets the patient, both have in mind some kind of conceptual model of the patient's internal system, however complete or incomplete that may be on either side. We all know that doctors think in terms of nervous systems and circulatory systems and digestive systems and so on; most psychiatrists, psychotherapists and psychologists think along similar lines (although they may deny it) of real or imagined shifts in neurophysiological functioning, brain biochemistry, of psychodynamic complexes, structures, mental constructs and defence systems, of built-in repertoires of thinking (cognition) and behaviour, any of which may be assessed, evaluated and then treated.

The external system is even more elaborate. It is about the kind of person the clinician is, the nature of the relationship with the client (partly in the heads of both, partly outside), the whole machinery of the encounter from the status (real or imagined) of the clinician and the clinic to the equally part-real, part-attributed qualities of the patient and his or her background. It is even about the setting in which they meet and what the labels on the letterheading and the look of the place convey, or are meant to convey; this includes whether or not the latter is conducive to what doctor and patient are trying to do. It is about the real-life effects on the patient of, for example, a troubled partner, a stressful job, a bullying peer group, strains in school or college or in the culture or subculture; and it is about the kind of effect all these external realities have on the clinician too; his or her immediate colleagues, or people in other services whose help may need to be called upon; about training, supervision and support; about everything from the most elusive influences such as 'image', attitudes, myths and realities about healthcare, feelings, esteem and clarity of the job one is supposed to be doing, to such down to earth matters as time management, space, and whether the tools for the job (like the telephone system) work in a way which helps or makes things worse.

All this, I believe, is as relevant to what goes on in the clinical encounter and to every kind of therapy as the material identified as 'internal'. But it is very hard to think about; in fact it is very nearly impossible, and there is always the problem that when subjects are so vast and complex we tend to introduce specialists and special language (jargon) or, even worse, acronyms. These protect us from thinking even as they set out to clarify.

We tend to look to the core differences between specialties (e.g. surgery, psychotherapy, social work) rather than look for areas of connection; we set up journals, academic departments, exams.

It is bound to be that way, now and probably forever, and the point of the dual clinical/systems consultation described in the following pages is emphatically not some kind of all-embracing theory of how it all works or how it can all be made easy, but a multipurpose toolkit for finding a way though all this, and trying to illuminate the scene.

The usefulness of systemic consultation

- As a joint exercise in looking at what is wanted, what is needed and what is possible, and in assuming that the consultee has more to contribute than even the consultee might have thought, it puts any shared enterprise on a surer footing. Whether as colleague or as client, the consultee has a solid role.
- The focus on the *autonomy and responsibility of the consultee* (again, as fellow professional or as patient) tends to keep the problem near to where it started out. A problem in school remains with teacher and parents, instead of being reassigned as a clinical case in a children's clinic. This may or may not reduce waiting lists, but it will certainly make possible a more rational response, for example by a consultative visit by a psychologist to a school rather than a child being simply booked onto a six-month waiting list for a two-hour assessment that it turns out isn't needed. This in turn makes space in clinics for people who do need specialised assessment and treatment; what happens via systems consultation is that the criterion of needing specialist help is not only in the clinical signs, but in the answer to the question 'how much can the front line people (patient, family, front-line professional) do for themselves, or at least contribute?'
- If this makes sense then you will see that a consultative 'valve' all the way down the line (e.g. parent to teacher to school doctor to specialist and on to other specialists), at each step exploring what may still be possible at each step despite anxieties for a change, can reduce the number of people involved and supports continuity of care. Many treatments fail not because they're wrong but because they aren't used properly, monitored carefully and persisted with.
- There is a cost in providing such consultative steps but it is a reasonable hypothesis that the introduction of consultative steps would save time and money. Consultation could also help make sense of waiting lists.
- *Very* importantly, it is a joint learning and teaching exercise, consultant and consultee (colleague or client) knowing more for next time, for the present problem or for other problems. Clinicians end up knowing more about their colleagues and their patients (and their respective settings)

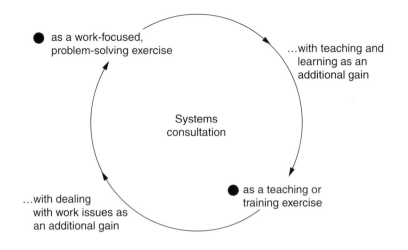

Figure 1: Circular relationship between systems consultation in training and as a work-focused exercise.

than they did; patients learn hands-on healthcare, self-care and about prevention, linked to matters close to home. Such learning is problem-focused, that is to say the problem came first. But one of the attractions of the consultative approach is that it operates just as well the other way round: as teaching or training focused on day-to-day problems. Consultative approaches may therefore be arranged, or sought, primarily for problem-resolution, with hands-on learning as a 'bonus', or primarily for training, with problem-solving as the secondary but important gain.

- The consultative process allows for the irrational and emotional (e.g. loss of confidence in persisting with a particular approach, or anxiety about asking for an explanation or an alternative) and trains those who practice it in practical empathic understanding; good intentions are not enough. The competent consultant must be genuinely curious about how and in what kind of environment the consultee functions, or tries to function, and against what odds. At the same time, respect for the other person is not about being polite, but about sifting through and actually negotiating openly what each is thinking about what the other can take on, about whether they can, or how much they can, and what help is needed. This goes both ways in true consultation, and a good test of 'proper' consultation is that role-reversal for a particular reason should not be a problem.

- Given this kind of collaboration, with every question and doubt admissible, it is difficult to see how bad practice, bad behaviour on the part of patients (now perceived as equal partners, not irresponsible children), mutual ill-feeling, complaints, enquiries and litigation would not be significantly reduced.

Complications

The complexity of healthcare seems to have taken us all rather by surprise. The Golden Age of Medicine – always the day before yesterday – was simpler, as myths are. Doctors had wisdom and authority. Indeed, the less they could do, the more wisdom and authority was attributed to them. Nurses and perhaps a secretary did their bidding, unless the doctor was junior and the nurses very senior, when the question of who was in charge was reversed. There was something of the archetypal family in the practice or in the hospital – the wise old buffer, sometimes gruff but always kind, supported but kept in check with discretion by matron; and the youngsters, the junior doctors and nurses, working hard but having fun, cheeky and frivolous in their default settings, but capable of earnestness, indeed melodramatic seriousness, at the appropriate times. Other professions were hardly visible, though somewhere behind the scenes there were helpful magicians in the laboratory, the pharmacy and the x-ray department. Administrators, from the governors to the porters, were anxious to be of help, and, lest we forget, there were the patients too, whose chief attributes were gratitude and respect and, often, being interesting cases. And that was it, really: you had a pain, the doctor weighed it up and prescribed something for it, and you got better, worse or died. This may be a caricature and mythical state of affairs, yet an examination of even the most modern medical soap operas suggests that these archetypal ghosts still haunt the medical places.

Something has happened to medical care since. Chapter 4 is an attempt to outline some of the reasons for there being so many minefields and disaster areas on the horizon. For the moment, here is a list of some prominent problems on the contemporary scene, particularly those which consultative approaches might be able to help with. My shortlist has 13 main categories of problem.

1 Traditional authority – anybody's – is no longer clear, and where it is clear it is neither automatically nor universally accepted.
2 Technical authority – that based on knowledge and skill – tends to be subject to controversy and challenge.
3 The relative ownership of rights and responsibilities are in a muddle, and this causes anxiety, resentfulness, suspicion and defensiveness.
4 Different members of the medical team have different and sometimes imperative views about their relative authority, rights, roles, skills and responsibilities. This can cause conflict.
5 There is in healthcare a need to be, to seem and to feel competent and in control, while the realities of healthcare largely operate against this. The psychological impact of this tends not to be acknowledged.
6 The high-speed advance of health science is producing unlimited possi-

bilities and at the same time, true to the integrity of science, as many admitted uncertainties. Thus all the facts are provisional.

7 This high-speed advance makes constant learning necessary and makes 'best practice' also at best provisional.

8 The kind of science that we and many scientists are familiar with values objective models (the statistical manipulation of closely defined, large scale data and primarily *linear* conceptual models – page 32) which are at odds with the complex, fuzzy-edged, multidimensional, intuitive, value-driven (e.g. ethical, cultural), subjective and a-rational kinds of information needed to complete the full picture of health, disease and treatment.

9 All this, from ambivalence about authority to the explosion of different kinds of data, increases the pressure for ever-increasing specialisation, which is in turn institutionalised by professional examinations, certification, expectations and career paths, and by our organisations, journals and teaching and conferences.

10 Despite doubts about medical solutions to health problems (and to many less well-defined problems in living), demand continues to expand faster than it can be met. This expectation comes from policy makers as well as the population, and is shared, enthusiastically or otherwise, by many practitioners. It is not a bandwagon to jump from, either for doctors, patients or governments. The whole world wants it, too.

11 The irrational in healthcare is not adequately dealt with. A skeptical public still want magical solutions. Doctors denying being omniscient and omnipotent nevertheless can be drawn into colluding with this fantasy.

12 All this is amplified, sometimes grossly so, by high levels of information, misinformation and controversy, much of it immediate and with journalistic 'angles' rather than considered and reflective, and much of it contradictory, coming from the publishing and broadcasting media and other forms of information technology.

13 Just as medical scientists bravely and helpfully try to get at the hard facts 'within' all this, as if the rest can be put to one side, policy makers and managers try to manage it all as if more money, more working parties, more policies and action plans will get the beast under control. This 'top-down' approach has shown no signs of justifying its cost.

Given the contribution of such things to uncertainty in medicine, the short definition of consultation is worth revisiting: a jointly undertaken exploration of what is wanted, what is needed and what is possible.

Consulting with the reader: is systems consultation possible?

The account so far is of mounting and daunting complexity in healthcare systems, plus a tale of the benefits of using the relatively new and perhaps unfamiliar techniques of systems consultation to deal with it. Snake oil practitioners, of course, build up the problem before reaching into the covered wagon to produce the cure. Is it possible that the treatment is worse than the cure? That systems consultation, especially locked onto clinical skills, amounts to just too much to bother with? Even more complexity, and worse, new complexities, perhaps ones the reader hadn't thought of, or considers irrelevant. Might the cure be worse than the disease?

The truthful answer is Yes and No. In the preface I suggested that in dealing with highly complex systems useful, pragmatic simplicity is achieved only *via* a journey through complexity. Consultation taken as a whole does have its own complexities, though perhaps more in what it reveals than in how it proceeds. On the other hand, the implications of what the consultative process uncovers can be complicated, and also not always clinical, not always welcomed, and not always soluble. I believe several of the examples illustrate this, and I will sum up some of this – where consultation impinges on policy-making and politics – in the closing chapter. Some may be rather taken with the idea of systems consultation and wish to make it central in their own work. But it could also be useful as an accessory in day-to-day work.

Elaborate though the explanations and underpinnings of consultation are (Chapter 3), doctors for example do not have to remember all the anatomy in Gray, every nerve, blood vessel, muscle, ligament, bone and length of gut in the body, and how they go under, over, through and around every organ. Probably many competent doctors who would not now stand a chance of passing a basic 1st MB anatomy examination nevertheless, faced with a patient with, say, back pain, can sift through all the right diagnostic possibilities, probably faster than they are aware, because of the anatomical groundwork they once did. The same applies to much of medicine, and other fields too. Having once learned the basic stuff means an almost unconscious scanning and ranking of the possibilities, whether the presenting problem is a headache, a backache or rising damp. I would like to feel the same could be true of systems consultation; that one could become familiar with the *kinds of system* that operate outside the individual and which colour the whole of assessment and treatment, and the ways in which systems consultation clarifies these things – indeed, points out they are there at all – and ways of working with them. Further, that this familiarity could also become second nature, so that it informs the clinician's style of work without adding more time to the clinical consultation than it

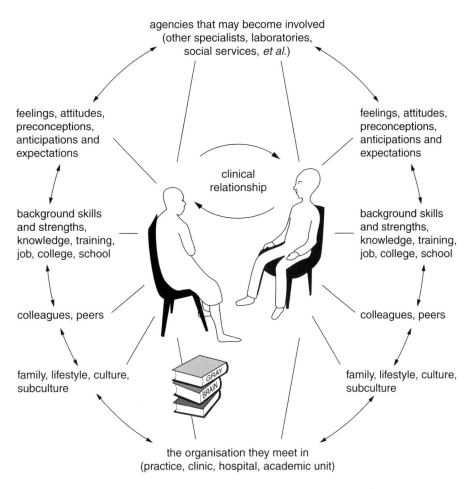

Figure 2:   The wider external systems.

saves. Whether it can, and does, would perhaps be useful to research. My assumption is that even if it did make some consultations longer, it would be likely not only to save time overall, but make work more interesting and save energy too. Taking peripheral distractions and moving them to the centre of the frame can be a surprisingly interesting move, converting frustration into curiosity. As the early biologists pointed out: irritability is the first sign of life.

The rest of the book

Chapter 3 is a more detailed account of systems consultation and its variants, and Chapter 4 discusses further the inherent complexity of health-care practice and services, and why it is likely to get more so. Chapter 5 gives examples of various applications of systems consultation in medical work and in Chapter 6 examples are given of consultative principles applied in working with groups and teams. Chapter 7 focuses on systems consultation in relation to teaching and training, and Chapter 8 is an exploration of using systems consultation alongside clinical consultation as a natural partnership, evaluating the inner world (literally and metaphorically) of the patient's system alongside the outer system. Chapter 9 is a discussion about how the experience of consulting systematically and thoughtfully with others, advances the capacity to think through one's own work and decisions, in crises as much as in longer term matters. Chapter 10, the twist in the tale, proposes that such consultative approaches provides a route to our patients becoming equal partners in healthcare. Chapter 11 is about areas of cross-fertilisation between consultation, narrative principles and the humanities. Chapter 12 contains some conclusions. You *could* try reading it first.

CHAPTER 2

What are we talking about?

- Defining some terms.
- Internal and external 'other' systems in healthcare.
- Kinds of conversations in healthcare.

The terms in the title

Complexity and *systems* have already been outlined. By *medical care* and *healthcare* I refer to the work of all in the healthcare fields: doctors, nurses, clinical and educational psychologists, different kinds of healthcare practitioners and therapists, and those who manage their services. I appreciate that not all clinicians think of themselves as 'therapists' and many therapists would not consider themselves clinicians. I use these terms variously in the book, and no doubt inconsistently, as with 'he' and 'she'. The same applies to the use of 'patient' and 'client', though possibly there is some justification in using the former term for someone receiving clinical services. 'Client' has become popular in recent years but, like 'customer', doesn't quite hit the right note.

A note on the medical model

For the purpose of this book, I see its professional readership as having in common a primarily *diagnostic* approach, based on their understanding of the internal physical and psychological systems and perceived needs of their clientele. I take this to be the hallmark of the much discussed and much criticised 'medical model', even if what is diagnosed by the expert professional is a faulty diet, wrong thinking, disturbed feelings, something in the environment affecting them within, or showing patterns of troubling behaviour. I would suggest that *this* – diagnosis of B by A using A's expertise – is the essence of the medical model, rather than the assumption of physical

11

causes (Tyrer and Steinberg 2005; and page 151). Systems consultation is its antithesis, as I hope will be clear from the account in this book. Both are important, and overall, within healthcare, each complements the other.

External and internal systems

The 'other' side of medical care is partly within, as the *psyche* and one's repertoire of behaviour. However, different people do conceptualise the psychological dimension in rather different ways. My own assumption about human psychology is that it is a dynamic system understandable from psychoanalytic, behavioural, neurophysiological and relationship perspectives, and that to subtract any one of these dimensions is to subtract something from the reality of the whole person (Tyrer and Steinberg 2005). 'External' relationships are hard to disentangle in psychological and psycho-somatic terms from the outer material world and the way it is perceived from within; being comfortable with reciprocally interacting systems is a help. I would say that the spiritual is important too, but as a concept it loses as well as gains by being elusive and understood in different ways by different people. Whatever else the spiritual refers to, I think it also encapsulates something about the totality of the person, including hopes, wishes, the creative imagination and as a sense of the aesthetic, all of which seem to me vital in human evolution, development and functioning rather than optional extras (Steinberg, forthcoming).

The external components of these interacting systems are those to do with the people we live with and those we work with, either close up in our teams and practices or in other departments and agencies elsewhere, and this is mirrored in the equivalent networks of contacts and relationships of which the patient is a part. The ethos and atmosphere will be determined by many group and organisational influences and pressures, but also by cultures and subcultures which may be, for example, to do with such things as socio-economic class and background, ethnic group and professional norms and expectations. Even in the supposedly 'one-to-one' consultation there are likely to be rather influential 'ghosts' present, for example representing the network the doctor is embedded in, and the family network the patient is embedded in too. And of course they can be ghosts of Christmas past, as well as Christmas present. It can help to be aware of this. Also powerfully influential are matters to do with information, attitude, ethics and the law.

Then there are things like appointments lists and timetables. Systems are not only to do with the way things develop between people, but what contains the whole process, the 'three Rs': rooms, rotas and resources. Sometimes consultees seem as unaware of how deficiencies in such things are undermining their work as they would be of 'interference' from the unconscious. As some of the examples show (e.g. Example 6, page 82), work problems for which people sometimes blame themselves turn out to be caused by not having the proper tools for the job in terms of space, time and material equipment, such as a quiet room and comfortable chairs.

Such things, from the nebulous to those that are down-to-earth, constitute this 'other' side of medicine.

Different kinds of conversation

Why 'the *language* of consultation'? Although this book is full of methods and strategies of systems consultation and even offers some rules, I am suggesting that in a more general kind of way there is such a thing as a consultative way of doing things – a consultative style of conversation. It is a dialogue between equals, as far as the task in hand is concerned, with no assumptions or preconceptions about the outcome, because if there were, the consultee wouldn't be asking and the consultant wouldn't be trying to help the consultee find out. The notion of a 'consultative style' may seem rather vague, but I suggest that other kinds of interaction – for example the ones systems consultation is contrasted with on page 15 – do carry with them a whole set of assumptions to do with the attitudes and expectations of the participants, the respective status of each, their relationship and the way they talk and listen to each other.

For example, at the core of a *clinical consultation* is the interview of B by A; perfectly reasonable teachers and books refer to it as the 'interrogation'; it is about questions – a preset list of questions which students learn and which the patient doesn't initially know about, nor about their significance. It is followed by the examination, both physical and to a greater or lesser extent of the patient's mental state.

Although *psychotherapy* sometimes begins with questions (as in clinical work, 'taking the history'), many psychotherapists primarily *listen*, on the basis that asking questions brings up what is important to the therapist, while what should come up are matters on the patient's agenda. This may seem to veer somewhat towards the consultative approach, but isn't, because, however tangential the approach of the psychotherapist, it is about gathering information about the patient's inner world and trying to make sense of it in the therapist's terms.

Characteristically, many individual and group therapists are prepared to sit silently and non-committally as the minutes tick by until, with rising tension and dissipating defences, the patient feels moved to say what matters. The caricature of the psychotherapeutic approach has the patient sitting in silence with the therapist perhaps gazing out of the window or, if trying to help, possibly raising his or her eyebrows in a friendly and enquiring way from time to time. The patient finally asks, 'what do you want to know?', to which the reply is: 'what do you want to tell me?' (Lest the reader unfamiliar with the ways of psychotherapy thinks this can only be a caricature, it is worth mentioning there have been studies looking at the pros and cons of explaining to patients in advance about how the sessions might be conducted, and that sometimes describing how psychotherapy proceeds is positively helpful; but many disagree.) It also needs to be said that systems consultation, or training in systems consultation, is conducted by some trainers and practitioners on the basis of generating group feelings which the consultant feels should be worked with. My own view is that this tips the balance of the work away from using the consultee's own understanding and towards that which the consultant wants or needs to use. However, it will be found in some areas of consultative work and training.

I hope this conveys how a psychotherapy session might come across to an observer. In contrast, a consultative session would sound like a conversation, and needs to be one. Caplan (1970) has said, for the benefit of the novice in the consultative field, that if the would-be consultant were simply to listen while the consultee recounts at length the story and details of a problem and then asks 'so what shall I do?', it is very unlikely that the consultant would be able to reply with anything useful.

A *supervision session*, where a trainee or junior is reporting to a senior colleague, will also have an atmosphere of its own, and whatever the style of supervision there will be the expectation of some kind of more or less systematic report to the supervisor, who will indicate what's alright and what's not, and who will encourage, warn, advise or explain as appropriate.

Teaching can be consultative in style, and as will be seen, one of the strengths of systems consultation is that it is a joint learning exercise. However, prescriptive didactic teaching has its key place in education, and as every schoolboy knows, it does not sound like consultation.

A problem we have in terminology is the use of *supervision in teaching and training* which is distinct from *administrative, hierarchical supervision*, but may nonetheless involve the latter, e.g. a senior doctor supervising the work of a junior. Such supervision may also include both didactic and consultative-style teaching. An additional problem of terminology is that training in psychotherapy is commonly described as both 'supervision' and 'therapy'. All the consultative approach can offer this hazy area is to acknowledge that it *is* unclear, rather than deny it, and when the issue comes up, to follow consultative guidelines and ask: what's actually happening? Who is doing what with whom?

Liaison work, where different professionals or units collaborate (e.g. Huyse 1997, 2000) may involve any combination of advice giving, case sharing or consultation. Finally, support may be a useful side effect of consultative work, as of good training and good administration, but is not a primary aim of consultation.

To return to the kind of conversation that consultation is, how might it sound? Obviously, not like someone instructing or checking up on another,

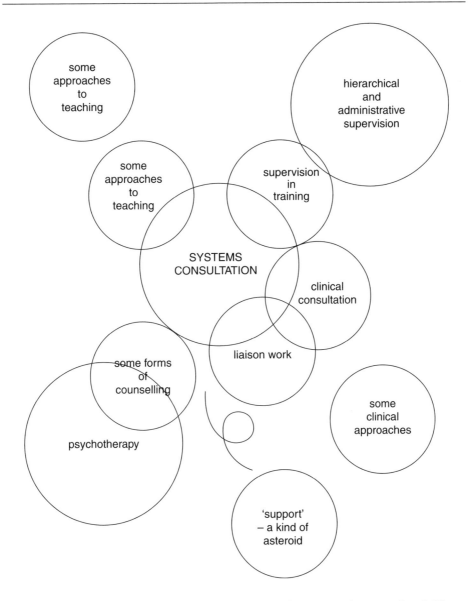

Figure 3: The consultative universe: activities similar to, touching on, overlapping with and different from systems consultation.

and it would not usually have either the long silences or expressions of challenge or concern of psychotherapy. Nor would it come across as someone of higher status talking to someone of lower status; there would be neither words of reassurance nor approval. Rather, as implied, it would be conversational, and informal but focused and businesslike, with no inhibitions by either side about making sure the work stays focused by reviewing progress and purposes and clarifying points – especially uncertainties about terms used. We all use jargon, but no mysterious term should be allowed to pass unexplained and 'on the nod'. As mentioned earlier, the special language of consultation is plain English, and that is quite innovatory enough.

CHAPTER 3

The key to complexity: systems consultation

- A description of systems consultation.
- The aims of systems consultation.
- Practicalities: time and place and who takes part.
- Different kinds of systems consultation.

Putting the cart before the horse

I am going to describe systems consultation before saying more about healthcare's chaos and complexity (in the next chapter) because the kind of instrument of enquiry that it is says something about what it is up against, just as we could tell quite a lot from, say, a boat, a kite, a tractor or a rock drill about the kind of environment it is designed to get through.

It is important to appreciate that chaos isn't intrinsically a bad thing, but a new way of understanding systems that are so complex they don't obey our known rules (e.g. Gleick 1987; Burton 2002). At the same time, recognition of the inherent complexity and incipient chaos of healthcare systems provides us with an opportunity to widen our understanding of the field, just as quantum theory has increased our potential to understand physics immeasurably beyond what was understandable in terms of the Newtonian physics we learned at school. It is not as if all is well in healthcare; new paradigms to supplement the old are timely. Just as Foucault said of psychoanalysis that for all its deficiencies it at least 'made possible a dialogue with unreason' (Foucault 1967), so systems consultation provides us with some practical ways of negotiating chaos and complexity.

Defining systems consultation

The basic unit of systems consultation involves one person, the consultant, helping another, the consultee, to describe a problem or issue in his or her own words, using the concepts and methods of his or her own professional work. The consultee remains autonomous in that work and responsible for the matter that is being discussed. To repeat the earlier mantra, it is a joint, peer–peer exercise in finding out what is wanted, what is needed and what is possible.

This definition contains a number of important implications for this kind of consultation. For each, to fill out something of the 'flavour' and ethos of systems consultation, I will show (a) how it differs significantly from other kinds of consultation, and (b) where it can go wrong.

The consultant does not diagnose the situation, still less diagnose the consultee

The consultant's job is to find out about the consultee's work, situation and any problem or issue described, not to tell him what it is. A revealing test on contemplating a piece of work as consultant is whether you are genuinely curious about what you will find, or whether you go in with a preconceived idea to start out with. It is only human, and perhaps necessary, to go in with a kind of set of provisional models for what may be found, and in any case some such set of templates is likely to grow with experience. Nevertheless, the most important single quality the consultant should take into consultation is curiosity, and it follows that consultant as well as consultee should learn something new from the consultation: the consultant something useful about the consultee's work, the consultee something useful about the process of consultation and how it widens his or her understanding and perspective.

1 How does this differ from clinical consultation? Because here we need the clinician to know more about the nature of the problem than does the non-clinician, and to detect and assess it by the clinician's own knowledge of symptoms and signs.

2 What can go adrift? It is a reality that many people offering systems consultation will already be experienced and probably relatively senior in another field and will be used to being relatively controlling, inclined to be paternalistic or maternalistic, and quite often frankly bossy. Correspondingly, some consultees in some circumstances may be tempted to let the consultant take over and say what is wrong. This can become a collusion, quite often powered by anxieties of one sort and another, and wholly or largely unconscious, so that the work reverts to a more atavistic, non-consultative relationship. Caplan (1964, 1970), one of the pioneers of this kind of consultation, and himself a psychoanalyst by training, commented that psychoanalysts had more trouble than most in working consultatively, being more familiar with questions about

motivation than behaviour (*see* for example page 36 *et seq*). The task in systems consultation is to clarify what is happening, not why (*see* Example 7, page 86).

The consultant does not supervise, still less take over, responsibility and authority for the matter in hand

The consultant relies on the independence and autonomy of the consultee, who agrees both to using the consultant's skills and to the subject for consultation. It is also for the consultee to decide whether or not the consultation has been useful and worth learning from. The consultant does not take over management of the matter in hand, nor responsibility for it.

1   Again, this is clearly different from the clinical or therapeutic situation, where the clinician's skills are needed for much or most of the problem. (But not *quite* all, for even a surgical operation needs consent, and the wider kind of consultation has a role here.)
2   What can go wrong? A great deal, as we will be seeing. For example, the consultant may believe he or she is offering this kind of non-supervisory, non-prescriptive consultation, while those authorising it may think the consultant is offering supervision. Such things happen, and can be potentially problematic (*see* Example 10, page 91).

Systems consultation is a peer-peer exercise

Consultation is not a cosy exercise in everyone being democratic, for example where, say, a senior practitioner or nurse takes a consultative-style training session with a group of junior colleagues or doctors and all sustain for the afternoon the fiction that they are all professional equals. If the session is consultative, the consultant's primary role and status rests on skills in keeping illuminate the consultees working situation and how they are equipped for problems and other issues that arise – problems in the 'other' side of medial care, not routine textbook matters – and how they are going to handle them using skills and experience appropriate for their status.

1   In didactic teaching the knowledge and opinions of the teacher are paramount: that's what the teaching session or lecture is for. Teaching on a consultative basis opens up the matters even the most experienced teachers might not have thought about.
2   Suppose the assumption is incorrect? That, for example, a consultee turns out neither able nor willing to engage in consultation, or having done so hasn't got whatever it happens to take to manage the matter under

discussion appropriately? This discovery is important for all concerned and the consultation has to handle it (*see* Example 8, page 88).

Systems consultation is conducted openly, with confirmation and clarification as necessary of where it is heading

As an exercise it is to be trusted, because, paradoxically, things are not simply taken on trust; everything is open, for review – for example, that a work problem which consultant and consultee thought amenable to a systems consultative response instead needs something different, perhaps more prescriptive. Anything should be made explicit if it helps the task of consultation forwards, even if it is the consultee's disappointment with the consultant or vice versa. It does mean that some sort of contract or agreement, its formality varying with what is being embarked upon, should be agreed at the outset. Further, it should be regarded as a strength of the procedure, not a flaw, if consultant or consultee calls a halt and expresses the view that things seem stuck or going off track or that a new focus for the work is needed. This is not a problem; as said elsewhere, it is what consultation is for. It takes skill to be a good consultee no less than it takes skill to be a good consultant.

1   In saying how this differs from much else in professional relationships, suffice it to say that it is not unknown for specialists to cover areas of uncertainty with mystification; that some psychotherapists value raising tension and 'useful' confusion in their clientele by ambiguity and silence; that some managerial meetings seem to a newcomer to be conducted in Mandarin Chinese; that some behaviour or levels of competence among professionals, and which we will describe here simply as hard to understand, are tolerated, sometimes for years and at great cost, from a mixture of embarrassment and lack of 'machinery' for tackling it. Consultation, ploughing on through perceived strengths and perceived weaknesses, designed to take everything in its stride with realism, courtesy, naive questions, and with its focus firmly on what's actually happening and the job actually being done rather than the personalities involved, is seriously different. If the consultee should wonder if such devices are getting in the way of work, *ask*.

2   Can anything go wrong, with such fail-safe procedures? The wheel can still come off the wagon, and the tendency to instability in all living systems, organisational and individual, can always come into the consultation as background noise and then as a force 8 gale. There is always room for surprises.

   Perhaps the commonest error is in not clarifying at the outset precisely what is on offer, intended and agreed, and hoping to patch up a flawed contract while going along (*see* again Example 10, page 91).

Aims of consultation

There are two things to consider here: first, the specific focus of the piece of consultative work, and second, whether the purpose of the consultation is primarily to help with an issue at work, or primarily to contribute to training.

The *focus* of consultation, to be agreed from the outset, may be:

1   a problem or question concerning the consultee's own clientele (client-centred consultation)
2   a problem or question concerning the consultee's work setting, which may include immediate colleagues or team, or the wider organisation (work-centred consultation)
3   a problem or question concerning the consultee's own professional functioning or development (consultee-centred consultation)
4   a fourth possibility, less of a routine and referred to above, is consultation-centred consultation: 'What's going on here?'

This focus may shift during the consultative process and if so, this should be made explicit (e.g. the consultant or consultee suggests it) and agreed.

Whichever of these is the focus, the overall aim of the consultation can, as said, be one of two things, either:

1   to help *handle a work problem, question or issue* or
2   as a *training exercise*, perhaps for the consultee's professional development or the development of the team or organisation, using a work problem, question or issue as the focus.

This reciprocity in consultative work was illustrated on page 5 (Figure 1), and is the key to understanding what the consultative process entails: learning from the consultation is one of its most important distinguishing features. (We do not always learn when simply shown 'how to do it', still less when the expert takes over.) However, whether systems consultation is engaged to deal with a problem or primarily as an aid to training depends on what is wanted, agreed and contracted for.

The time and shape of consultation

Systems consultation may be one-off, sometimes in a crisis, or a series of consultative sessions can be planned. Consultation may be between two people, or with a group. Consultation is portable; as a particular way of discussing work, two people ought to be able to consult with each other in the corridor or over coffee: but a useful outcome of a hurried ad hoc consultation may be to agree a better time and place for it.

As a style of conversation, consultation can also occur during another kind of meeting. For example, during a didactic session to use new equipment, a question may come up (e.g. 'could it be used for situation X?') which may be best served by switching to a consultative mode ('tell me about X').

Consultation can take place in the consultant's office, but there is much to be said for holding a work-focused consultation in the consultee's place of work. There is no hard and fast rule here: it is open to consultation.

Should a consultative meeting be minuted? I don't think each twist and turn of the discussion should be minuted, because that would be about its process, rather than its conclusions. A consultation whose aim is to reach a group conclusion or decision will probably want its conclusions and any future plans recorded in some agreed way. Another kind of meeting is less to reach a group conclusion than to help participants think something through. Each would then go off with their own personal ideas and feelings about how to use what they learned, and this might or might not include taking or proposing an operational or administrative step on their own – not the group's – responsibility. I think the latter kind of meeting is 'freed up' by not keeping a record. As to which kind of meeting it is – consultant and consultees can ask each other. *See* page 68, on notes.

Who takes part in the consultation?

The consultation should have a clear purpose, and the points made earlier are reminders that it is ultimately the responsibility of the consultees to achieve it.

Therefore those present are those able to decide and implement whatever emerges from the consultation. *See*, for example, Example 1, page 67, and Example 8, page 88. A quite common mistake is to consult with middle grade staff about how they handle their work (for example helping nurses develop their skills in dealing with relatives) and finding that implementation of these improvements become blurred with unit policies, which are beyond their remit. Another was identified by Caplan (1970) as 'mandated' consultation, for example when a senior member of the organisation (e.g. a head teacher) brings together a visiting consultant and a group of teachers the Head thinks 'need seeing'. This group may well not know why they are there, and may well misunderstand the purpose of the meeting and even resent it, especially if the visiting consultant is a psychiatrist or psychologist. Both situations contravene the points made on previous pages, break the rules, and are likely to run off the road.

Another issue concerns not only who has authority to implement whatever may emerge from the consultation, but who has the necessary information for useful consultation to proceed. Those with responsibility for making managerial decisions to deal with a problem or improve a service may have a mixture of statistics, hearsay and individual observations to go on, but a careful consultative exercise with them might well show several gaps in knowledge about what actually happens that only the front-line staff could supply. The unavoidable absence of the only person able to complete key parts of the story can apply to senior staff too, particularly where there is either a high level of overt anxiety in an organisation, or more covert anxiety about change. Senior people may be too busy to attend, or (as with other sorts of meeting) may find themselves only able to 'drop in for some of the meeting' (i.e. arrive late and leave early). It is not unknown for them to delegate someone to represent them, for example a short-term locum, or someone highly respected for their research role but not familiar with the organisation (*see* Example 5, page 79).

This does sound rather like blaming the absentees; however, those calling for a consultative meeting may themselves be responsible for giving the impression that what they really want is a kind of 'enquiry' with themselves as chief prosecution, key witnesses and jury; in which case the absentees' instincts may be right – that a joint, peer–peer exploration of an issue, with no prior assumptions about its conclusions, is not really what is wanted; in other words, not really a consultation as defined at all. It is because such insidious group pressures may be operating, probably only partially recognised if at all (and likely to be denied if pointed out), that the consultant needs to be alert to the psychodynamics of group behaviour even though not conducting group therapy. It is another reason for the invited consultant to hold a pre-consultation meeting to clarify the agenda.

Sometimes people who are keen to attend may not have the authority to deal with the matter for consultation. This particularly happens when different kinds of hierarchy meet at the point of consultation. For example, a local authority social worker consulting with a medical team about their joint handling of a child care case is likely to have very different line management from that operating in the clinical team. He or she might well expect to report back to a senior colleague, while the clinical team may be more or less autonomous. 'Reporting back' in this way would not be a problem for the consultation process, but it does raise the question whether the social worker's senior colleague should have been invited as well.

In summary, for a systems consultation to happen:

- The information expected to be available from the consultees must meet the needs of the agenda.
- The possible decisions to be reached – even if only to take a proposal to an appropriate committee, for example – must be within the capability and role of the consultees.
- Unless the consultative meeting is already a regular event, the invited

consultant should have a 'pre-consultation consultation' with those calling for a meeting to check (a) the above points, (b) what they understand by 'consultation', and (c) how they will communicate what the meeting is about, both to those participating, and to those who need to know the meeting is happening anyway.
- The consultant needs to be vigilant, and diplomatic.

All this may seem no more than common sense. But it isn't commonly found in health and care transactions, with much time-wasting and wasted energy as a result.

What's on the agenda?

The most important characteristic of everything that should be on the agenda for a consultative meeting is curiosity: not least curiosity about other people's certainties. 'What to do' about something is admissible enough, but 'how to proceed' is closer to the task of consultation. Thus, as mentioned earlier, if a definite decision is reached, that's fine, but more often consultees benefit from the very openness, honesty and uncertainty that enables them to then take an issue forward decisively in some way, in other aspects of their work and if necessary other kinds of meeting. This is why consultative meetings of this sort don't necessarily have to have a particular fixed place in an organisation's programme, although agreement may be needed for staff to spend time in that way. The effectiveness of consultation does not depend on having a position in an administrative hierarchy, but in the way it provides space, time and sanction for the consultees to think things through, together or separately. They may then be able to make personal decisions about their work that they otherwise wouldn't have reached. This could include decisions about how to use existing administrative machinery, or indeed to propose establishing new ones.

Thus the shared understanding within a team that a specifically consultative meeting could always be arranged, if people thought it useful, can be more important than giving it a place on the routine timetable.

The kinds of subject that characteristically emerge for consultation include:

- Client-centred consultation:
  - A nurse asks for help with a patient's case.
  - A school asks for guidance about a pupil.
  - A trained counsellor seeks regular consultative help in client management.
  - A general practitioner isn't sure whether to refer a patient to a specialist clinic or not; they discuss the options.

- Work-centred consultation:
  - A medical team keeps running into difficulties.
  - A unit is hit by a serious organisational or patient crisis.
  - A confident and effective unit wants to develop its work in a new direction.
  - A residential unit for disturbed children asks an outside professional to take regular consultative sessions with its staff.
- Consultee-centred consultation:
  - A member of staff has run into a difficult professional dilemma and asks for help in sorting it out.
  - A healthcare worker is wondering about a career change and would like to discuss it.
- Consultation-centred consultation:
  - Questions are being raised about the usefulness of a regularly held consultative group; the group allots a session to review this.
  - During a first meeting the consultant or consultee has doubts and wants to check whether the right things are being discussed.

(Examples in all these categories are given later.)

The story so far

I hope a picture is emerging of what kind of activity systems consultation is. To review this:

- It was developed as a set of strategies for helping professional workers collaborate, and this is relevant to helping healthcare workers operate together and make the best of their own and each other's skills amid the complexities of healthcare. It is identified as systems consultation here to distinguish it from other kinds of consultation, of which there are many.
- Systems consultation deals here primarily with the individual operating in his or her working environment, and its concepts and theoretical roots are in the psychological and social sciences and philosophy relevant to healthcare, including ethical questions.
- Clinical consultation, while being concerned with the above areas too, has as its primary focus the diagnosis and treatment of disorder. (It too deals with 'systems', of course, the internal systems of the body and the theoretical systems of the mind, but in this book the term refers to the wider range of systems than those which are, as it were, beneath the skin.)
- Systems consultation here is adapted to the healthcare setting by considering systems consultation as part of a dual strategy (clinical consultation being the other one) to help professionals engage with both clinical matters and organisational matters, especially where they overlap.

- In the foregoing (and hereafter) I have defined systems consultation fairly closely, with its own set of guidelines and rules, and with a list of other professional activities, which, variously, are very different or which overlap. A tool for dealing with the complexity and chaos to be found in healthcare systems should not itself be more complex or chaotic than can be helped, and needs a clear role and set of rules. It needs to be pragmatic and adaptable, and to function as a sorting and tidying up activity, for example to enable other meetings to be more productive. Some examples are given where failure to define systems consultation adequately – for example in an agreement or contract – can be risky.
- Systems consultation may be confused with hierarchical supervision, which it is not. Rather, it is a peer–peer exercise of jointly shared exploration of a question using the consultee's perspectives, not those of the consultant.
- Systems consultation is a learning and teaching exercise: the consultant learns about the consultee's problem and circumstances, while the consultee is likely to find out more about how he or she handles work and learns about the consultative process too. Both go away better equipped than they were before. This kind of consultative work is therefore a teaching strategy as well as a problem-solving strategy, and indeed may be chosen primarily as a teaching strategy.
- It takes competence and responsibility to be a good consultee.
- The way consultative work proceeds, that is as a conversation dealing with ways of handling problems at work and feelings about it, means it can resemble some aspects of some psychotherapies. However, the focus is the job, not the consultee's personality, mood or any real or imagined emotional problem, which is why it needs to be differentiated from a therapeutic activity. However, as the consultative work involves feelings and attitudes affecting work and the consultee's own self-management as a professional, both participants need to tread a careful line to make the most of psychological information and skills without slipping into psychotherapy. For example, *what happens* in work is the focus, not the consultee's motivation; if a consultee is, for example, 'depressed' about the work, the appropriate lines of questioning are about how this affects the job, and how the consultee is going to manage. Feelings of competence and control about work that result from a useful consultative session may make all the difference. However, suppose those depressive feelings persist, perhaps even making the consultation unworkable? In such a situation it would be a proper use of consultation for the consultee to see, or be helped to see, that therapeutic help for the depressed feelings needed to be obtained from elsewhere, to make doing the job (and using consultation effectively) feasible. That is up to the consultee.

(While on this point, the issue of *teaching* is similar. Consultation is a teaching and learning activity, as has already been said; but if consultation demonstrates areas in which the consultee needs to brush up his or her skills or knowledge or pursue further training, that can be a new decision for the consultee to make.)

Concluding note

Systems consultation is about systematically asking questions – clearly of course, respectfully it is to be hoped, probing if necessary, persistently, and with the expectation of straight talking on both sides. If what A says to B sounds muddled or a like a kind of personally or politically manipulative evasion, or if there is simply a lack of information that ought to be available, B should ask for clarification. And if in the end A is unwilling or unable to be straight and clear, and this leaves B with a problem that consultation is not going to resolve, then B can explicitly acknowledge this positively by asking: 'then where do we go from here? And when? At what time? And who will take the minutes?' A senior person being evasive about how he or she intends to resolve a controversial administrative matter (for example about the distribution of staff, or who is going to be on an appointment committee), and who is trying to take refuge in vagueness about the machinery ('I expect it will all be sorted out') might be asked something like 'how are we going to find out about this machinery?' 'Who do we need to ask about it?', 'Who's going to do that?', 'Shall we agree that now?', 'Let us know by when?' or 'Shall we fix the date?' This is an organisational enquiry, but the same kind of sustained questions may be appropriate for a vague or unanswered clinical matter, like a discharge date, or an arbitrary-seeming change of treatment. I mention such things not to encourage interrogation by consultation, but as a reminder that, nice and positive though consultation is, and generously accepting as it is of all the uncertainties in our work, it doesn't have to accept all that is woolly, and when appropriate can press for clear answers. Consultation is an exercise for grown-ups.

Menzies (1970; and Menzies Lyth (1988) demonstrates the amount of effort teams or organisations (in her reports, a hospital) could unconsciously devote to ensuring that matters for which the organisation was set up were not dealt with (*see* page 49). It is a common finding, in dealing with the problems of individuals as well as organisations, how much energy may be used in keeping a problem going, and how little is needed by comparison to make small, pivotal changes that can make all the difference. Finding the pivot point and what change to make is no easier in clinical work than in systems consultation. Systems consultation provides ways of asking questions to everyone's advantage.

CHAPTER 4

What seems to be the trouble? Why healthcare is complicated, and will get worse

- The components of complexity.
- Linear models *vs* systems models.
- Applying systems thinking to healthcare.
- Psychodynamic concepts and complexity.
- Narrative approaches and complexity.
- Attachment theory and complexity.
- Groups, teams and institutions.
- A healthcare dystopia?

> There are nine and sixty ways
> Of conducting tribal lays
> And every single one of them is right
> Rudyard Kipling, *In the Neolithic Age*

The components of complexity in healthcare: and why the problem cannot be stated simply

If a straightforward account of the complexities of healthcare was possible, it wouldn't be complex. The terms 'complexity' and 'chaos' identify multi-dimensional, dynamically interacting open systems which are inherently unstable and unpredictable, and characteristic of living, growing systems. While we may not understand the rules of chaos, perhaps we need quite different kinds of understanding. It may seem fanciful, certainly infuriating to some, that the intuitive understanding of intuition and poetry may in due course provide as important and effective a perspective on natural systems as mathematics, but Niels Bohr said as much, when grappling with the problem of how to convey his insights into quantum physics. Mandelbrot (1977) and his demonstration of the repetition of similar patterns in natural systems at every level from the smallest to the largest straddles the mathematical and the poetic, and we may need this kind of dual vision and integrated thinking to manage the intuitive and the objective in complex, natural, human systems like healthcare services. We tend not to.

Multidimensional doesn't mean merely that many factors are involved, such as hospitals, community services, self-help groups, alternative medicine and so on; it means that quite different concepts are involved too, for example very different kinds of theories – to select just a few: biological, pharmacological, behavioural psychology, psychodynamic theory, ethics, politics, economics, theories of management and philosophical questions such as what constitutes illness – *and* the myriad kinds of practice and controversies that flow from these. This alone is daunting, or ought to be.

Dynamic refers to different parts of a system – physical, social or psychological – constantly affecting and changing each other, so that the goalposts may also change. Perhaps the simplest physical example is a central heating system thermostat. As the sun sets, the temperature falls within the house and the radiators switch on. This will depend on such things as the house's insulation (including whether or not windows and doors are left open and the different position of the rooms). At a particular temperature a relatively simple physical device switches the heating system off, so that the radiator temperature drops; and at a particular low temperature the device switches the system on again. The system is therefore self-monitoring, and operates through what engineers know as feedback systems: the central heating system operates according to information about how it is doing out there in the room. Now, this is a simple system, but consider the many variables – and we haven't even touched on disputes between those in the house about where to set the ideal temperature. In the simplest social system dynamic a confident practitioner inspires confidence in her clientele, and this helps maintain the self-esteem of the practitioner. But what about ambivalent feelings and mood changes in the practitioner – the norm? That way lies chaos – also normal.

An *open system* is affected by matters from outside. Thus, our confident health worker is getting along fine with her clientele until she learns that her unit is going to be closed down. This kind of external influence makes the system unpredictable and potentially unstable.

A grand scheme for the totality of the healthcare system cannot be drawn up, but some of the conceptual models and bodies of knowledge which contribute to understanding it can at least be listed and outlined. That is what most of this chapter is about, after which there follows a short account of why things can only get worse.

Casting a wide net

The following subjects can throw light on different aspects of healthcare systems and why they are chaotic and complex:

- complexity and systems theory
- psychoanalysis and psychodynamic thinking
- from psychology to myth: narrative approaches and consultation
- psychodynamic concepts applied to groups
- groups, organisations, institutions
- value, ethics and the humanities
- accounts of what it feels like to be a doctor, and a patient.

A major contribution to the complexity of healthcare is that there is a great deal of controversy about diagnoses, including the status of some diagnoses and indeed whether they exist at all, and much the same dispute about treatments. Some of the supposedly mutually contradictory theories, particularly in psychology and psychiatry, in reality are due to mutually contradictory and conflicting theorists and practitioners; opponents of a particular perspective tend to characterise it as rigid and extreme and then dismiss it. In fact – as anticipated in the Kipling quote – many of these variegated theories all have their place in dealing with different kinds of problem in different ways, and many which seem quite different are perfectly compatible with each other. There is no intrinsic incompatibility between, for example, psychodynamic theory, behaviour theory, neurophysiology and neuroanatomy. Some of the latest findings in neuroscience demonstrate this (e.g. Damasio 1999). Most of us have minds, brains and bodies and use all this equipment when we develop problems or make use of treatment; as pointed out earlier, therapists may be superspecialist, but as patients we tend to be generalists (Tyrer and Steinberg 2005).

None of the brief notes that follow represent a complete picture, even in summary, of each area; rather, it is intended simply to convey the different kinds of way one must think in order to comprehend the different kinds of contributions to complexity in healthcare. There are some references for further reading, but remember the point about Gray's Anatomy on page 8; the point is to be aware of the contributions to the healthcare kaleidoscope, and correspondingly the kinds of issues that may be operating around a focus for consultative work.

Remember also that what follows only represents the non-clinical, 'other' half of the story. The internal systems of a human being, those that constitute the focus of clinical consultation, are quite complex enough in their own right; we borrow the psychological factors for the purposes of this account, since, as we will see, the *psyche* will not be pinned down, and (fortunately for ourselves) straddles the inner and outer worlds.

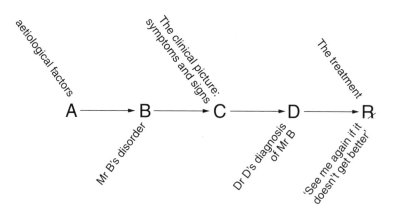

Figure 4: Linear model of aetiology and intervention.

Complexity, and linear versus systems aetiology

Earlier (page 30) the point was made that different models of under-standing are useful as the keys to different kinds of problem. An engineer designing a bridge will use Newtonian physics about mass and gravity, while a nuclear scientist will employ quantum physics. In healthcare, the *linear explanation* that aetiology A causes condition B and that therapy C will put it right is economically satisfactory (economical in the intellectual sense as well as in terms of cost) for a great many conditions. However, the linear model is inadequate for description when more things have to be taken into account; for this, the systems model is more appropriate. Burton (2002) summarises the key components of a complexly interacting system in the following way:

1   it has multiple components
2   these components interact unpredictably
3   they are influenced by their initial state
4   they are influenced by their environment
5   the interactions are non-linear, that is to say, there is no simple 'A causes B' relationship (e.g. 'high cholesterol levels cause heart disease', supposedly) but the outcome depends on the state of the system's components at any particular time and quantitative and qualitative aspects of each part of the system
6   action or behaviour emerges (emergent behaviour) that cannot be predicted because it is qualitatively different from the components of the system, and from what the system has done before and
7   complex systems are open; once observed, the observer becomes part of the system.

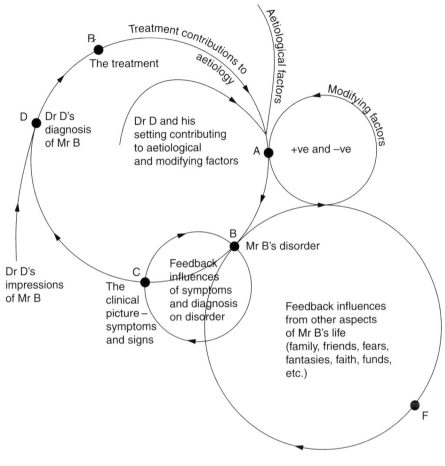

Figure 5: Systems model of aetiology and intervention.

Complexity and systems theory in healthcare

When we are stuck for an answer, it is always worth considering that we may not be asking the right sort of questions. Asking the right questions about modern healthcare has taken quite a long time to develop, and meanwhile the whole culture of medical care has changed too (page 58). The wider healthcare issues that are now taken for granted require that the old linear models of explanation need supplementing by systems models.

New ideas take a very long time to filter through, however. For example the bold new science of quantum physics, with all its extraordinary findings about what waves and particles seem to do, began around 1900 – about the time Freudian theory was beginning to make its mark.

Systems theory has its roots in the same era. Every medical student knows about Claude Bernard and the concept of homeostatic mechanisms that maintain the *milieu interieur* (1857, quoted in Sukkar *et al.* 2000), just as equivalent self-correcting systems in machines were understood and engineered, for example James Watt's steam engine, in the eighteenth century, and various kinds of thermostat ever since. The anthropologist Gregory Bateson gives an interesting account of the application to living systems of observations made on machines, notably by the nineteenth century physicist Clark Maxwell. He was asked by engineers to provide some kind of formula on which to base blueprints for reliable steam governors, themselves internally self-governing systems like the thermostats described on page 30. The engineers had found that their machines, and by implication their theories about them, didn't always work, despite looking as if they ought to work, on paper. (You would have thought so: steam pressure rises, engine speeds up, the centrifugal governor whizzes round and rises up a column, and at a certain height cuts off the steam, thereby slowing the engine; whereupon the governor moves down again, and back comes the steam pressure. Simple enough.) Clark Maxwell, however, showed that the nature of the internal structure of the device was not enough; what mattered for the device to work was not only its timing, but also the timing as affected by entirely external events, for example if the steam machine with its governing equipment was expected to start trundling uphill, or to power another piece of equipment. The puzzled engineers were thinking only of the internal design of the governor, but what mattered were the timing of events around the governing circuit and their effect on each other, *and* the interaction of all these events with what was happening outside the circuit, i.e. what the machine was doing or how it was being used (Bateson 1979). A more complex kind of simplicity was needed – one that *included* the other relevant factors.

A distressed member of a family seeing someone in the healthcare team in a large clinic represents a more complex system than a machine stalled at the foot of a hill; yet it was something like a 100 years before what was learned from nineteenth century engineering problems began to have impact in health clinics. This began with the emergence of family group therapy, probably beginning with the clinical work of John Bowlby (Bowlby 1949), the biological work of Von Bertalanffy (1968) and the anthropological and psychiatric studies of human communication by Bateson and his colleagues (Bateson *et al.* 1956; Bateson 1973, 1979; and see historical accounts in Gorell Barnes (1994) and Bloch and Harari (2000).

The basic assumption in family therapy is that the origins (and therefore potential for therapy) of the presented problem (e.g. a depressed parent or an anorexic or misbehaving child) are not only in the presenting patient, but in the family system of which he or she is a part. Now, this is not the place to go into the complexities and controversies of family therapy, which boil down to how much of some clinical problems and their treatment are best understood in this way. As a clinician I would say that there must always be *some* family interaction (e.g. the effect of one family member's heart attack, cancer or depression); that sometimes (I am referring to psychiatry here) the whole of the problem and the whole of its management is best understood and most responsive in the terms of family therapy; yet also that, very often, whatever the mixture of coarse and subtle mutual influences from various systems (e.g. family, endocrine), some conditions are most effectively understood and treated individually. I would recommend reference to the comprehensive accounts of family therapy by, for example, Gorell Barnes (1994) and Bloch and Harari (2000). As Gorell Barnes points out, the systemic model of human feelings and behaviour that developed in the study of families is extendable to the wider social systems involved, too, for example schools, health services and other organisations. While major developments in systemic models derive from studies of work with families, one may apply the term 'systemic' to a whole range of organisations involving people interacting with each other. This is taken further in discussing organisations (page 50).

Practical implications for systemic consultation

In some respects family systems therapists and people engaged in exploratory consultative work approach their work along similar lines. Broadly:

1   prior and reasonably precise agreement about what is wanted by the clients/consultees is sought.
2   attention is paid to (i) who is responsible, and able, to describe the nature and ramifications of the matter in hand and (ii) who is in a position to do something about it. They are expected to be involved and invited to the assessment, typically by inviting to the clinic 'everyone living at home'.
3   as clinicians and therapists, family therapists will tend to think diagnostically (despite perhaps being ideologically hesitant about doing so) but the problem is ordinarily converted into something the family should handle. Thus a referral of a child with 'behaviour disorder' (the supposed responsibility of the clinic) is metamorphosed into misbehaviour which the family, led by their parents, is expected to deal with.

But suppose that they can't. For example, marital discord or some other reason for the parents not being able to agree a consistent approach to the child is quite common, in which case the focus appropriately shifts to trying to deal with that, or perhaps suggesting marital counselling as a precondition of continuing with family therapy. Or, the child may seem to have problems that don't respond to improved and systematic parental handling, in which case he might need individual assessment for (for example) attention-deficit hyperactivity disorder (ADHD). In each case the serial questioning and serial hypotheses of family therapy, exploring with the family what *might* work, can lead in due course to the demonstration that something else, more individually and clinically focused, is needed. The situation is the family therapy equivalent of the systems consultation finding in Example 6, page 82 – that the anxiety of the consultee, a counsellor, wasn't due to a 'disorder' or an aspect of her personality but arose from aspects of her work that she hadn't thus far recognised. Thus systems consultation acts as a kind of filter, differentiating what basic, front-line (and often commonsensical) advice will be sufficient if persisted with, from those problems which become defined as needing a more specialised approach. In Chapter 12 we will review such 'discoveries' of systems consultation, and see how placing it early in the referral system (instead of simply fixing an appointment with a specialist) could shift problems back from specialist care to generalist and even 'ordinary' common sense care (even self help) – but *with* the help of consultation, not as a kind of benign neglect.

Psychoanalysis and psychodynamic thinking

With the world of psychoanalysis and psychodynamic thinking we are in another universe entirely, and one beset from within and without by controversy. I will try to outline the essence of psychodynamic thinking and the kinds of model the psychodynamicists use.

Sigmund Freud founded what he called *psychoanalysis* during the nineteenth century, and the subject was taken further by those who broadly agreed with him, despite argument and schism (for example CG Jung, Anna Freud, Melanie Klein, Alfred Adler, and many others) and the wider field is generally identified as *psychodynamic theory* or *depth psychology*. Psychodynamic theory postulates that our wishes, attitudes, feelings and behaviour are powerfully influenced by psychological processes of which we are unaware – hence the *Unconscious*. We can become aware of unconscious influences and pressures to a helpful extent (i.e. achieving *insight*), but the depths of the unconscious can never be fully plumbed. Moreover, they supposedly go 'down' (because the model is in a sense layered, like geology – hence 'depth psychology') beyond what may be described in primarily psychological terms, to very primitive feelings and impulses which are as much animal as human, and particularly to do with life, death, love, aggression and sex. More than is sometimes realised, Freudian psychodynamic thinking is both biological and evolutionary in its account of the origin of such feelings. It is also a *developmental model*; that is to say, one that is understood as gradually taking shape as part of growth and maturation.

Jung's particular contribution to the psychodynamic model of thinking was to widen it out to include the influence of the *cultural*, *mythical* and *anthropological* history of the human race. Further, he invoked the important and controversial notion that humanity, as a vast group, shares the potential for such mythical figures and events embedded in its unconscious mind – hence the Jungian notion of the 'collective unconscious', the unconscious predispositions to form these inner images being known as 'archetypes', for example, hero figures, villains, magicians, wise old men and women. To some, such notions are not only nonsensical but rather scary, as if Jungian theory acts as a Trojan horse to import magic and mysticism into psychology. To others (myself included) a perfectly rational case can be made for the possibility of such phenomena (i.e. not necessarily 'true', but feasible) via evolutionary theory (e.g. Stevens 1982; Steinberg 2004a and forthcoming). I mention this controversy here (indeed, so controversial that one side tends to dismiss or deny the other and say there can be no argument) not to set a hare running but to remind the reader of the contribution of the Tower of Babel story to the grand complexity of healthcare. It is a real phenomenon in our institutions.

Back, however, to Freudian theory. Three well-known components of psychodynamic thinking are the *Ego*, the *Id* and the *Superego*. The Id is the primitive, unconscious beast within. The Superego is the name given to the outcome of the Id having to come to terms with the requirements and constraints of society: the 'conscience', more or less. The Ego is the sense of personal self and personal beliefs and values that represent a working compromise between the demands of the Id and the constraints of the Superego. Note that the Superego is – like conscience – a restraint within; and yet it derives from outside, from group (e.g. family, social) expectations. This 'taking on board' something from without is known as *internalisation*, as when the members of an institution (e.g. a team, a profession, a corporation, a nation, or a religion) adopt within themselves as second nature something from without. Another 'mechanism' – there are many, making up psychodynamic theory – is *projection*, where something an individual is uncomfortable about within (e.g. hostility, dishonesty, whatever) is unconsciously attributed to other people or groups. Another mechanism of which psychotherapy makes much is the *transference*, familiar in popular fiction as 'falling in love with the therapist'. What it actually means is that while working closely with a psychotherapist the patient transfers to the relationship feelings that belong to other relationships. For example, someone who has depended heavily, perhaps ambivalently and in an immature way, on other people may begin to be dependent in an immature way on the therapist. The problem in the patient's story then becomes part of what therapists call the 'here and now', right there in the consulting room, and available to be worked on. There is *countertransference*, too, that is to say, the feelings the psychotherapist develops for the patient. Psychotherapy training uses the understanding of feelings in the countertransference process; for example, feeling protective towards a patient may say something important about the patient (and the clinician) and reminds the psychotherapist to be aware of not falling for a manipulative pattern of behaviour (being dependent and seeking overprotection) that others in the patient's background have fallen for and reinforced.

One of the charges levelled against Freudian theory and its derivatives is that it is like a religion, stuck in the late nineteenth and early twentieth century and unable to move on, a charge inconsistent with the evidence. In fact one of the most interesting developments of psychoanalytic thinking began when Bowlby and his associates linked it to family groups on the one hand and primate studies on the other. The basic science of this combination is *ethology*, which is about what observed behaviour is for, in terms of what it achieves for the individual, the group and the species. Bowlby's theory, rather a set of ideas and theories, is known as attachment theory, and is discussed below (page 45).

Taken together, psychodynamic theories represent an elaborate open system, much of it largely or entirely submerged in the unconscious, and those who are prepared to accept its role in human behaviour must fit this most complex and ultimately unknowable, truly chaotic aspect of individual and group behaviour into all the other complex systems described here.

A short interval: who's who in psychological care

Not everyone is familiar with how psychodynamic theory fits into professional work. As this is very complicated indeed, and widely misunderstood, I will try to deal with it here in the interests of trying to encourage clarity in complex situations.

Psychiatrists (who are medically trained) and psychologists (who are not) *may or may not* train further in psychotherapy, and therefore become *psychotherapists* too (or *counsellors*, if they trained in counselling). On the other hand, there are other routes into training as a psychotherapist or as a counsellor, and social workers, nurses, indeed anybody regarded as having the academic, intellectual and personal requirements of the various courses, may train in psychotherapy or counselling.

Any of these workers may practice individual therapy, group therapy or family therapy. If their practice is informed by Freudian (or Jungian, or Kleinian, and so on) thinking, they would be regarded as *psychodynamic psychotherapists*. If they went the whole hog to practice the original, Freudian, highly specialised form of psychodynamic psychotherapy called psychoanalysis, they would properly be known as *psychoanalysts*.

Art therapists' and *drama therapists'* training combines art (or drama) and psychotherapy training. Many *psychologists* go into all the fields mentioned above, but many regard psychodynamic theory as either unproven or simply as nonsense, and favour *behavioural psychology*, that is to say, with their practice based on observable behaviour rather than assumptions and inferences about unconscious processes. *Cognitive therapy* (in full, cognitive behaviour therapy or 'CBT') is similarly behavioural in its approach to assessment and treatment, and teaches its clientele how to challenge and handle conscious ideas and attitudes that make them anxious or unhappy, e.g. ideas about not being as good as other people, or about the need to check and double-check things they do, as in obsessional disorder. There are also significant differences in training, and often the approaches, between *educational* and *clinical* psychologists, whose practical training is primarily in schools and in hospitals, respectively.

Should you want to read more about psychodynamic theory, Brown's slim account (1961) is still one of the best, Wollheim's on Freud is excellent (1971), while Sulloway's biography of Freud (1979) gives an important account of the ideas as rooted in biology. Stevens (1990) and Storr (1998) both give excellent and readable accounts of Jung's theory. I will also mention Hinshelwood's remarkably clear account of one of the most interesting yet inaccessible of the psychoanalysts – Melanie Klein – for those who are tempted (Hinshelwood 1994), because Kleinian theory is used by Skynner (1975, 1989) to throw light on some peculiarities of teams in organisations.

This is why I have gone on at some length about psychodynamic theories. Feelings of which we aren't fully aware, or whose origins we mistake (e.g. wrongly blaming X for them) come into psychotherapeutic relationships like risen ghosts. It is reasonable to assume that they, or something very like them, come into other relationships too: for example, between healthcare worker and patient, and between professional workers. This is inconvenient, adding enormously to the complexity of life, but I think it is a reality, and that allowing for it can make some sense of certain patterns of thinking and behaviour in our colleagues, our patients and ourselves which nothing else can explain.

Practical implications of the dynamic psychotherapies for systems consultation

Dealing with the non-obvious

I will say a little more about dealing with the psychological depths here, because this is what the 'other' side of healthcare involves. Much of what we feel about aspects of our work is irrational. However, as that term implies a kind of madness, we may prefer as a description for much of what goes on in providing and using health services the term 'a-rational' (= makes no apparent sense).

It is not irrational for a patient and a doctor, or one healthcare worker and another, to feel considerable warmth or great anger for each other, or both, because when human beings are intimately engaged in emotive tasks, especially for substantial lengths of time, such feelings tend to be generated beneath the surface. They are usually handled in the way all civilised people handle such feelings, by keeping them in perspective, by denial (a normal defence mechanism), by telling jokes to let off steam, and so on. Other feelings in the normal range common among healthcare workers are guilt, typically about 'not doing enough', self-doubt, anxiety and even a sense of danger (Steinberg 1991) and sadness, disappointment, resentment, paranoid feelings and, occasionally, even euphoric feelings of doing a good job. All such feelings, (including euphoria) can influence work, and the ways in which they arise from and affect work can be handled sufficiently by consultation focused on work. The principle that emotional problems can be handled by proxy is recognised in mature human relationships, in which consultation and some forms of psychotherapy may be included, where not everything needs to be said or hammered home. For example, the consultant may acknowledge the maturity and sense of the consultee by recognising that the latter's account of problematic competition with a colleague does not need 'interpretation' of personal or background issues that could hypothetically be contributing to it; identifying the matter, putting it on the table so to speak, should be enough, and if it isn't, that too will be apparent if 'competition' continues to be a work issue. This is not to pussy-foot around a difficult subject, as it might be in psychotherapy, but simply to remain true to that principle of consultative work which assumes competence on the part of the consultee who, given the time, space and atmosphere in which to explore things, will come to his or her own conclusions. (But suppose something like this, interfering with work, cannot be resolved in this way and a more direct approach is needed? *See* Example 7, on page 86). Finally, everything learned from psychodynamic theory and practice may apply as much to the consultant as the consultee.

In heading this section 'Dealing with the non-obvious' I am thinking not only of feelings which, as already said, may not be dealt with directly, but of the *consequences* of such feelings. For example, a domineering senior may inhibit confrontation from others because that is the way human groups (and other primates) keep the peace; the unspoken, if not unconscious, anxiety is that there could be a mighty row if X is challenged and that will affect the integrity and capacity for work of the group. The consultant, however, as naive outsider, can simply enquire (for example) whether a particular work decision is going to be reached by a single person's assertion or by discussion; and if so, how dissenting points are ordinarily made in the team.

Timekeeping

Although there are as many psychotherapies as there are drugs in 'MIMS', and they are all different, a common expectation is punctuality: stopping as well as starting on time, a courtesy which plays an important part in establishing boundaries and trust. Informality is fine, but the participant who arrives at a consultation meeting late or leaves early (or both) may be illustrating avoidance of the issue, as well as wishing to establish how many more important calls there are on his or her time. Such things are relevant in consultative work.

Confidentiality

Confidentiality is taken for granted in psychotherapy, and is important for consultative sessions too. In consultative work it is more difficult to maintain because the work tends to deal with the institutional aspects of personal issues, thereby referring to identifiable places and teams, quite often in a group. Not gossiping about a consultation outside the meeting is important because the consultative session has been set up specifically with the right people and the rules of engagement to tackle something, and continuing the debate elsewhere may be at least unbusinesslike and at worst evasive.

   As far as keeping records is concerned, it is the consultees who represent the points of reference, not their clientele or places of work.

Mystification

In this respect consultation should differ completely from some of the ways of psychotherapists. Caution in being critical is appropriate here; but some schools of psychotherapy do seem to foster (unconsciously of course) a degree of mystery (a) because the way they deal with things cannot be put into words, (b) because the way the therapist might explain something intellectually (including what the session is 'for') may not be how the patient would put it, and it is the latter that is crucial for therapy to progress, (c) because a certain amount of silence and ambiguity on the part of the therapist raises tension in the patient or group, which supposedly gets more efficiently to what needs to be expressed, and (d) because what the patient imagines the therapist is like, or may be thinking (as part of the transference) is more important than what the therapist is 'really' like, or 'really' thinking. As this is not a book about psychotherapy I won't discuss this further here, except to say that a consultative session should be the opposite in all respects: as discussed in Chapter 5 (*see* page 64), what the consultative session is for should be discussed and agreed, and how it and its aims and methods are perceived on both sides should similarly be open to discussion.

Thinking the unthinkable and saying the unsayable

The idea of the psychotherapeutic session as a time and place for discussing what cannot be discussed elsewhere is valuable for the consultative meetings; the latter is then treated as a special occasion for standing back from work to consider it.

Discussing work problems in a group may help sort an apparent total impasse into more comprehensible if not manageable components; for example aspects which have been, so far, difficult (perhaps merely embarrassing) to bring up, matters for which the 'normal channels' aren't clear, or things which might be achievable via a different strategy; the 'impossible' hard core may then turn out to be small enough to handle.

Embarrassment can be a very powerful obstruction to change – the established practices of institutions rely heavily on it. The opposite is also true: embarrassment can make it difficult to challenge changes that others claim to be desirable. In general, people tend not to want to be thought naive, foolish, ignorant, awkward, troublemaking or, worst of all, crazy. Even being thought conservative, radical or revolutionary can be inhibiting. People can be remarkably self-censoring, something which contributes powerfully to holding crazy institutions together, and institutions, in both the concrete and abstract senses, can be extraordinarily enduring and resistant to change – much more so than troubled people, and far less adaptable. A consultative session, especially in a group, may valuably provide an arena where saying what is ordinarily unsayable and rehearsing different ways of putting it becomes possible. For example, an angry member of staff may ventilate annoyance in the group relatively incoherently and inconclusively, then be able to work on his raw (though quite possibly appropriate) feelings later to think through how best to make the point, and to whom. Thus: feelings are acknowledged alongside keeping on track, with the task of useful, operational decisions being the eventual outcome. Similarly, a consultative group can help consultees sift through randomly expressed observations that would not get far in a committee, and help select the most usable, translating what is wanted into what is politically feasible. Ideas can also be put into rank order, or an apparent impasse can be transformed from something complex and indigestible into 'bite-sized', manageable pieces. If this sounds rather like advocacy, that's because it is; helping to articulate that which the consultee wants to say, but isn't sure how to.

From psychology to narrative and myth

Like many new ideas, the current importance of narrative in psychology, psychotherapy and social science represents the rejuvenation of something which is as old as the human race: the telling of stories. The traditional myths – how the world was created, tales of heroes and villains and so on – were the only truths we had until science came along with its own partic- ular brand of mythology, the 'scientific fact'. However, science's funda- mental integrity as demonstrated by the scientific philosophy of Popper or the evidence of quantum physics (e.g. Penrose 1990; Popper 1999), has also showed how 'facts' are provisional and the foundations of knowledge not as certain as they once seemed. I think it is true to say that the human mind, whatever else it does, is driven by the need to make sense of things, sometimes on inadequate data: hence our capacities for paranoia, fantasy, story-telling and creativity. We make sense of ourselves and our surround- ings, driven no doubt by all sorts of fears and wishes, but woven around such 'facts' as we have to go on. The cultural anthropologist Joseph Campbell nicely described myths as public dreams, dreams as private myths (Campbell 1974). We make some kind of story about ourselves and our lives or there would be no point in getting up in the morning. Even the hard-headed, completely rational scientist (another myth) has to have some such rationale for heading each day for the lab.

The idea of narrative sits uncomfortably with the idea of being objective, and is therefore completely consistent with the postmodern scepticism discussed briefly on page 54, and with the idea in social science of – to use the title of a classic book on the subject – the social construction of reality (Berger and Luckman 1997). Thus a narrative is someone's story, the account he or she constructs about themselves, their lives and their under- standing of a given situation, and we see them all the time and every day, in newspapers, broadcasting, books, lectures, scientific papers, the cinema and all other kinds of fiction. Taking narrative as simply someone's account of a particular view of reality, rather than that reality having a self-evident authority of its own, is an uncomfortable ideology, getting behind the scenery, so to speak, and questioning it. It applies the integrity of science to considering the scientist; the 'objective observer' operating a microscope is himself put under the microscope. However, while postmodernist decon- struction could be taken as being iconoclastic and destructive, narrative represents the other side of the deconstructive system in that it always allows for an alternative story.

Practical implications of narrative for systems consultation: it ain't necessarily so

Similarly to deconstruction, the process of systems consultation questions all assumptions, but the process also encourages other narratives, about problems and the components of problems as well as the possible solutions; its only ideology, to the extent that it has one at all, is 'it ain't necessarily so'.

The concept of psychology as narrative fits between theories of individual psychology and of group psychology because the individual's account of himself, even if only to himself, represents a gathering together, suitably collated and edited and rendered suitable for presentation to others, of an autobiography (McCleod 1997). Working on people's stories puts consultation (Steinberg 1989, 2004), psychotherapy (e.g. White and Epston 1990) and general practice (Launer 2002) into a position where people are helped to look again at what they have *made* literally of themselves and their predicaments and in a new questioning, creative light consider revision or even a rewrite (as I have suggested elsewhere (Steinberg 2000b), the role of the psychotherapist as editor).

In systems consultation the myths that may need rewriting could include the consultee as being responsible for everything, or incompetent, or powerless, the unhelpful colleague as potentially helpful, something which has 'never' worked as possibly working this time, and so on. It therefore combines pragmatism with encouragement to find out and to experiment, initially with ideas, and then in practice. If something 'doesn't work' the narrative to be discouraged is that it 'can't work' and the storyline to be encouraged is *how much* it has not succeeded and how much it has.

Earlier, the consultative process has been described in terms of putting things into shareable, understandable words: plain language. The idea that the primary purpose of language is to communicate may be essentially true, but to communicate *what*? There are plenty of circumstances where language can be used to communicate several things, e.g. to placate, reassure, dissemble, divert, impress, intimidate, and so on, and this is not unknown in the workplace or between therapist and patient. By using ordinary words, unlike technical jargon, institutional assumptions and the rhetoric of alleged 'correct' opinion (all of which belong to technical, traditional or self-appointed authority), negotiation becomes possible; where the conduct of the conversation is in plain language – consultation's *lingua franca*, and often an alien tongue in academic, technical and managerial circles – everyone is on an equal level. The remark about the meeting conducted in Mandarin Chinese (page 20) was not entirely frivolous; this was the language of the Chinese managerial class, as was the use of Norman French in eleventh century England.

In some circumstances, for example in looking at team and organisational development, it can be interesting to use even more basic 'language', for example that of drama (de Haan 2004) or painting (Steinberg 1989a, 1991), to get below, so to speak, all kinds of fixed assumptions in order to take a really fresh view. Examples are given in Chapter 7, and in a later chapter we will look at the contribution the arts and humanities in a more general sense, as encouraging means of communication which are shareable in a way that technical language is not. It is important to remember that all this is not in aid of dismissing whatever this or that technical authority maintains; it is because a difficult or insoluble problem has a considerable authority of its own, namely that which cannot be done, or even thought about. It is the authority of problem maintenance that systems consultation, working its way along with questions and answers in plain English, sets out to query, working on the hypothesis that the narrative of the problem is, often enough, a significant part of the problem.

Psychodynamic thinking applied to groups

In an essay *The Large Group in Training*, (1975) Skynner, psychotherapist and staff group consultant, described phenomena familiar to people who work with groups: that ideas, attitudes, feelings and behaviour ordinarily associated with individuals can appear as the predominant, emergent mental climate of a group. A group, like an individual, can seem unsettled and uncomfortable, then 'in more than one mind' as different members make different kinds of progress, there can be moments of euphoria when whatever the group's task happens to be seems clear and attainable, and times of group depression when things don't look quite so good; at difficult times there can be paranoid stages, where the group sees itself as entrenched against outside elements that don't or won't understand it, won't help, or even threaten it. In Skynner's account he drew an analogy between Kleinian theory (e.g. *see* Brown 1961; Hinshelwood 1994) where the infant is thought to proceed through a *paranoid stage* (an external world 'peopled by Gods and Demons' – the ideally good and the completely bad) to a *depressive stage* ('greys' rather than black and white) which is more mature. Many adults and leaders of groups would be able to recognise in themselves and in their teams times when everything seems impossibly against them, generating anger and blame, particularly towards the outside world, and later more sober, reflective periods which represent neither blame nor self-blame but a realistic appraisal of what is difficult and what is feasible.

As Kipling recommended in his well-known poem 'If', 'triumph' and 'disaster' were both imposters to be rejected by the mature adult which I mention as yet another reminder of the replication of enduring ideas within the culture and of the common themes in the heads of people, groups, organisations and across activities and professions too. This perhaps should not surprise us, and yet pointing out the similarities across physics, biology, psychology, organisational theory and the humanities can seem quite novel. All these things are produced by similarly constructed brains.

Attachment theory

I will enlarge on Bowlby's attachment theory for four reasons. First, because it deals with the interaction between psychological systems 'within' and those without, i.e. intrapsychic dynamics and the dynamics of group relationships. Second, because it is consistent with several psychodynamic concepts which contribute to understanding how groups of people function. Third, because a key concept within attachment theory is the idea of *a safe base from which exploration is possible*, and as we shall see this is a relatively straightforward and relevant working model for consultative work. And fourth, because its commentary on how higher primates relate to each other, which helps root our model firmly down to earth, happens also to have a bearing on what we see in healthcare systems, as I will explain.

Attachment theory (Bowlby 1969, 1973, 1980; Holmes 1993) is actually a system of ideas and hypotheses rather than a single theory. The basic attachment dynamic (*see* Figures 6 to 9), like a Mandelbrot fractal (*see* page 30, Mandelbrot 1977; Gleick 1987) and interestingly rather like Blackmore's self-replicating cultural ideas (Blackmore 1999), is in its basics relatively simple, yet capable of replication at different levels of organisation, and into more elaborate versions of the same basic pattern. For example, it makes sense at the level of observable interaction between individuals (Figure 6), as a 'memory', though more an incorporated experience (Figure 7), as a thread in the adult repertoire of behaviour in relationships (Figure 8) and similarly as one method of feeling and thinking about demanding or merely expectant people – who of course are similarly equipped themselves. Thus: through evolution, child development, personality development and group relationships in four consistent steps.

Attachment theory takes the compelling evolutionary position that the primate infant could only survive in the jungle and therefore reproduce by having the following innate capabilities:

- to have ways of recognising and keeping close to a protective adult
- to elicit caring behaviour from the adult
- to explore its environment and survive the experience.

These three, proximity-seeking attachment behaviour (A), care-taking behaviour (B) and exploratory behaviour (E), are preconditions of surviving and developing a normal, adaptive life, and are held in a self-regulating dynamic system. (Of course, the adult has to be capable of care-giving in the first place, but we are then involved with higher-level attachment theory, where the successfully growing and maturing infant has grown up to become an adult capable of looking after infants.) The absence of a protective, nurturing adult, the inability to elicit the latter's attention, unwise exploratory behaviour (e.g. into the jaws of a predator or over a cliff) or too close clinging to the parent could all upset the system, and provide explanations for childhood and parental problems seen in everyday practice such as neglected or overactive, risk-taking children; except that we are not in the

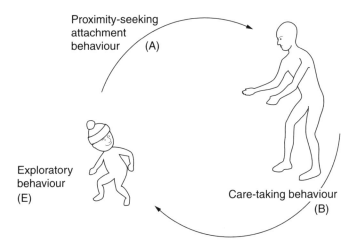

Figure 6: Attachment dynamic: actual patterns of behaviour.

jungle – though it is a useful metaphor – and have various surrogate, educational and therapeutic ways of helping.

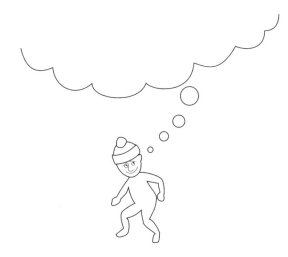

Figure 7: Attachment dynamic: continued internally as experience.

The experience in the real, external world of a sequence of parenting experiences that were 'good enough', to use Winnicott's commonsensical yet sophisticated term (Winnicott 1972) then becomes part of the developing infant's own maturing, capable state; it has, within what Winnicott called the facilitating environment provided by the parent, 'taken on board' or 'introjected' (*see* page 37) the good experience of being able to cope, and becomes confident, capable, able to explore safely and to handle human relationships. To use another metaphor, the child develops 'backbone'.

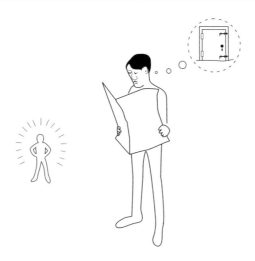

Figure 8: Attachment dynamic continued: past experience now influencing adult parenting skills.

We have here a narrative (a kind of evolutionary myth, if you like) that is consistent with adult emotional problems too; people who are overdependent, or high risk-takers, for example. To give the story of the basic model another twist, however, even the most mature and capable of adults under pressure can revert to an earlier step in the maturational chain (reversion to what used to work: like a tantrum). For example, if an overdependent, demanding patient pesters me for long enough for a remedy I cannot provide, even *I* might become angry and impatient and (to use the psychodynamic term) regress to a less mature way of handling a distressed patient. If pushed, I might communicate my own discomfiture to a colleague, who (if he or she is capable, and I have communicated in a reasonably mature, professional way) may well be able to help. Or, I might be regressed enough to get angry and refuse to treat the patient; though there are of course more sophisticated, institutionalised ways of avoiding problematic clientele. (Figure 9) Thus the attachment model, beginning millions of years ago in evolutionary terms, or within the lifetime of the individuals in ontogenetic terms (i.e. personal development), can provide a viable explanatory model for dysfunctional behaviour in relationships and in groups. Similarly, it provides a model for ways in which patterns of help-seeking and responding (or not responding) can be communicated throughout teams and organisations in a kind of emotional/behavioural chain reaction.

The kinds of feelings aroused in professional workers and that can make the response to our clientele err towards the negative do not have to be obvious and extreme like overt anxiety and anger. For example, to avoid anger or anxiety particular kinds of patients, particular colleagues, problems or even ideas can be avoided or ignored. Fear of failure is common among healthcare workers, who are characteristically self-selected for being

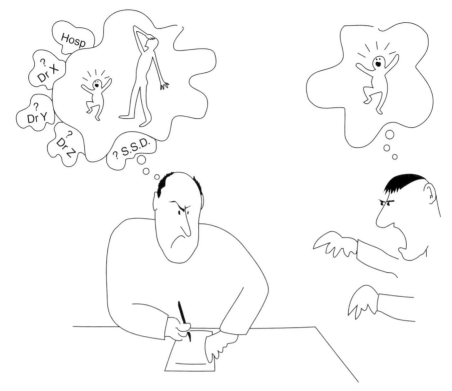

Figure 9: Could the attachment dynamic be influencial in the consulting room?

conscientious people who are motivated to help but may be neither person-ally, nor through their training and supervision, prepared for what this involves (Steinberg 1991).

Experienced human beings can see trouble coming, and we can arrange work and work settings with baffling systems (in both senses of the term) that minimise such encounters and experiences arising. It is not unknown for awkward issues (like impending death) to be passed down the line from the medical consultant (who cannot be seen to fail) through the senior nurse, middle grade doctor and then to the junior nurses, who may be perceived as too inexperienced to help adequately, something the patient will be aware of. Thus the problem seems to evaporate, except of course for the distressed patient and for the junior member of staff who goes home feeling guilty.

In the classic study mentioned on page 27, Menzies (1970) described how an organisation, overtly dedicated to caring, can maintain social systems designed to do practically the opposite, by a culture of the denial of feelings (those of the patients as well as those of the front-line staff), and by a policy of disconnecting and depersonalising patient and staff as individuals, by elaboration of rituals involving tasks and routines, by moving staff around and explicitly discouraging 'overinvolvement', by dealing with problems by reassurance ('you can manage', 'pull yourself together', etc.), by removing decision making from individuals by spreading responsibilities, and by supporting this dissipation of real care by paperwork, checklists, 'reviews' and other procedures; also by the politically familiar delegation of 'ultimate' responsibility upwards to people well away from the scene, and downward towards the most junior and inexperienced staff, whom even the patient might not expect to cope. It perhaps needs to be said that the hospital which Menzies Lyth studied was a distinguished one, and brave enough to have practices examined which were practically universal in hospitals, and no doubt still are, half a century later.

Some practical implications of psychodynamic and attachment theory for systems consultation

From psychotherapy in general, and adopting the guidelines of attachment theory in particular, an important criterion is that the group feels safe – a safe base within which to explore ideas and feelings and to have disputes – and control of this is shared with the consultant. Starting on time, stopping on time, stating explicitly why they have met and that the meeting is confidential, and using language that can be shared by everyone, are all part of making a clearing in the institution which feels like a safe base.

Sluzki (1999) has summed up a number of ways in which the consultant, by his or her style and behaviour, can help forward the task of determining what's happening in the group and its parent institution and enabling the consultees to play a full part in developing solutions. It should be reflective, that is to say willing and able to stand back from the task (including the consultative process itself) to see 'where we are getting'; it should be transparent, with no mystery about what is going on or withholding (or appearing to withhold) special knowledge about the group or theories about the group – Sluzki mentions in this context that the consultant should be fully engaged and working with the group, not aloof; curiosity is crucial – the group is finding out things together, not making any prior assumptions about a particular hypothesis about the problem or the solution being the right one; and there is an assumption of good intent – the consultant encouraging the group to see what is positive in the contribution of each member, without this detracting from the contribution of others.

Groups, teams, organisations and institutions

A group is simply a term for several people gathered together, and could be a fortuitous gathering, but for the sort of group discussed in this book there is generally an assumption of some kind of relationship between the members and some kind of common purpose. I would suggest that a group becomes a working group when it has developed a common purpose, ways of proceeding and various roles have been allotted or adopted, and by then it has some of the makings of an 'organisation', though this term usually implies that such things have been formalised to an extent. When an organisation, small or large, has developed a little history and an ethos, this is more what we recognise as an institution, although our culturally defined institutions usually require enough history and ethos to have impact outside themselves; in narrative terms, not only does the institution have its own story but others develop stories about *it*.

For completeness, I suppose a 'team' can be defined as a working group with an overriding set of objectives: like a team of horses, they are (or are supposed to be) pulling in the same direction with a particular end in mind, and in institutional terms a team will often be operating one of an institution's subsystems, including of course its direction and management. Among the most relevant to our discussion of working with systems, these groupings have in common to a greater or lesser extent:

- aims, real, alleged or imagined
- routine ways of operating plus other capabilities
- histories – which include changing, connecting with others, declining
- an ethos – a distinctive character
- ethical values, taken for granted or explicitly claimed
- an internal structure: roles that allow authority and responsibility
- an external structure they belong to, usually a hierarchy
- some kind of operating system that probably is partly self-regulating, partly chaotic – thus its members, aims, methods, achievements and openness to new ideas may well vary
- time, space and tools. It is surprising how important these are for the group, yet how easily forgotten as a source of difficulty. As several of our examples will show, time management, adequate space and provision of the proper equipment for the job can take second place to team feeling and thinking, while deficient material resources and poor time management can be undermining and destructive.

As well as all the above that is overt and explicit, even to the extent perhaps of being written down (e.g. in a team leaflet), there is an 'other' side, either unconscious or not ordinarily thought about. By this I mean not only group psychodynamics such as those that make a whole group anxious, depressed, paranoid or manic, but also unrecognised social assumptions; for example, a group may have several 'bosses' – the formal authority of its hierarchical 'head', the technical authority of someone with special skills, the traditional authority, e.g. of the 'old guard', or the personal authority of a charismatic or manipulative individual.

All these areas represent just some of the features of our 'Gray's Anatomy' of the structure, relationships and function of organisations.

Aspects of institutional functioning and development

An institution – something instituted – may be deliberately set up, or come into existence gradually and historically, or both. The Royal College of Physicians, and the idea of a doctor, are both institutions; so are the Freud Museum in London and psychoanalysis. Institutions have a history, a purpose and involve more than one person, if only as speaker and audience. A few people meeting regularly for a drink, or for a group meeting, develop some of the characteristics of an institution. Thus, instead of the participants starting from square one every time they meet (e.g. asking 'what's on the agenda?' – for I wouldn't call most committees institutions) the ethos of the institution produces a kind of mindset as soon as you engage in it. This isn't accidental; the institution is something created to survive from meeting to meeting, something to remember from last time and anticipate next time. An institution devoted to the study of, say, evolutionary theory, or stamp collecting, doesn't have to be defined every time its members meet, although there may be rituals (e.g. a prayer, or 'what'll you have?') to remind those present of why they are gathered together. This is cosy, convenient, containing and quite seductive.

Institutionalisation, by definition, makes it easier to proceed with any business that fits the ethos, without further explanation, than to try anything different. People who make and respond to the rituals correctly are immediately accepted; those who don't will be sanctioned in various ways, for example by being thought mad. As this would be highly embarrassing all round and embarrassment is something to be avoided at all costs (*see* page 42), institutions develop more or less civilised ways of letting you know what kind of ethos they have and whether you would be happy with it. All this makes institutions very powerful, and even institutions supposedly set up for dispute (e.g. university departments) can set quite tight limits on the type and pedigree of new ideas they are prepared to allow entry to. This is understandable, because it allows limits to be set on curricula and allows more time and energy for specialist depth, if at the expense of breadth. However, it means that the introduction of new ideas, even for debate, is like the proverbial difficulty of turning round an oil tanker; and while the tanker turns, many generations of trainees pass through the institution without being open to other ways of thinking. The problem is that even when brave souls do cross barriers, as they do, we end up with hybrid concepts like, for example, 'psychosomatic', which, useful though they are, may divide as much as they unite; thus the idea of a truly new field, incorporating both *soma* and *psyche*, would be quite difficult for an established institution to handle.

What makes an institution different from other gatherings together, meetings and chance encounters is that their history and their purpose can at some point reach a kind of critical mass and then becomes something else, bypassing not only the aims and objects of the people who first set the institution up but the expectations and assumptions of many of its personnel. As Cooklin (1999) puts it: the individuals in an institution may develop, they may 'grow', their thinking may change, but the institution that was set up in the service of their original idea may not change, either with them or with the development of the original idea. He goes on to say that continuing association with the institution 'may become reified, turned into "a thing", and maintained for its own sake rather than for the needs of the task for which it was set up'.

Many institutions do acquire highly complex additional aims. Many hospitals with long histories going back to the 'golden age' of medicine were set up by philanthropic citizens to bring together the needy sick and doctors and nurses, at a time when it was very clear what the words 'disease' and 'treatment' meant. A visiting professor of social medicine once asked us, as a new intake of medical students, what we thought our illustrious hospital was now *for*. Still for 'healing the sick', no doubt, to the extent that it was clear what 'healing' and 'sickness' meant, but also important as an employer of large numbers of people, from porters to professors, indeed providing a gigantic career matrix for many people to develop in, and as an institution which contributed credibility, status and roles for its employees at all levels, all the way up to the Health Department and government of the day; and increasingly as a kind of disposal and dispersal system for some of its clientele.

All of which may sound a little negative, but when considering the image of institutions, remember that negative connotations may be no less mistaken than positive ones, something worth considering in the light of the human tendency identified in Kleinian theory (and by Skynner, in *Institutes and How to Survive Them* (Skynner 1989, in Schlapobersky 1989), to assign ideas, people or things to the categories 'good' or 'bad' too readily. Most things are a mixture of blacks, whites and greys. In many areas of the health and care services, for example, especially where children are involved, staff are seen (and see themselves) as 'good' – as the rescuers – and the parents, or one of the parents, can be identified sometimes unconsciously as 'bad' (Steinberg 1986a, 1987). When things go wrong it is the health or careworker who is then 'bad'. Systems consultation should therefore be non-judgemental once under way (but note the advice on page 89 about circumstances which make consultation non-feasible). In order to proceed, consultation needs to assume what Sluzki (1999) called 'good intent' all round, its task being to ask how far we (consultants and consultees) are doing what we say we are trying to do, rather than to make value judgements. Value judgements aren't irrelevant, but should be made when deciding about entering consultation and in considering what the consultative work clarifies. *During* the consultation, at least while continuing consultation is feasible, value judgements are generally as inappropriate as they would be during a surgical operation; they do matter before and after.

The social philosophy of organisations and institutions

Social theory and philosophy mirrors psychodynamic theory. Just as Freudian psychoanalysis maintains that people's feelings, desires and behaviour are driven by internal psychological processes of which they are unaware, social theory describes external processes which powerfully influence behaviour, attitudes and feelings without our being necessarily aware of it. The 'raising of consciousness' of the political activist is thus the socio-cultural equivalent of the psychoanalyst's aim to help the client develop insight. In both cases the idea is that if we know about such things we can make informed choices.

Anyone interested in the borderline and contrasts between madness and sanity, between illusion, misrepresentation and reality, and between common sense and ideology (which I suppose might well apply to anyone interested in systems consultation) might find the turbulent corner of social philosophy known as deconstruction (Lyotard 1992), notably that of its main exponent Jaques Derrida (Norris 1987), of interest. It is controversial, and near-incomprehensible to me, bearing a relationship I think to the court jester (page 160), and has fuelled any number of iconoclastic and fashionable angles for a particular kind of reductionist and narrow academic literary criticism, and which tends to read as 'anti-literature', with the art, magic and humanity gone and only the bare bones of a supposed political motivation remaining. In fact I wonder why I am recommending it. However, particularly in the writings of Derrida, I read into it the idea, central in systems consultation, that, in the words of the lyricist, (as said earlier) 'it ain't necessarily so'. Just as a physicist can sit on a chair whose solidity he quite properly questions for the purposes of scientific enquiry, or Freud could smoke a cigar (saying, famously, 'sometimes a cigar is just a cigar'), the deconstruction philosophy raises doubts about whether what seems to be definite is definite, and the alternative meanings and implications of words. I believe we are undertaking somewhat similar tasks in systems consultation: asking about what complex systems *do*, as opposed to what they seem to do; and just because it is difficult, if not impossible, to get at the 'facts' (living systems being chaotic), that does not mean we should not consider alternative possibilities.

This kind of socio-cultural enquiry is not in an entirely different dimension to psychology and psychiatry; theories of inner and outer reality are consistent with some convincing neuropsychiatric conceptions of the nature of consciousness (e.g. Damasio 1999), with the kinds of systemic model which attempt to make sense of the substructure of the relationships, institutions and organisations such as those involved in healthcare (e.g. Sweeney and Griffiths 2002) and with the highly complex psychodynamics of individuals and groups.

As a whole, all this is, I think, a valid complex model for a highly complex system. It would be hard to anticipate a serious model for the totality of normal and abnormal human functioning *plus* the systems we have for recognising and treating order and disorder to be less complicated than – say – the phenomena which govern the sea. The complex and chaotic effects of currents, undercurrents, crosscurrents, evaporation, wind and weather, freezing, the forms of the land and the sea bed, the effects of gravity *plus* how we use all this information – a fine mixture of marine lore, navigation systems, tide tables, timetables, shipping routes and all the details of marine engineering – are hardly likely to be more complex and chaotic than a model for the body and the mind and its external relationships.

Practical implications for systems consultation of social philosophies of organisational functioning

In his account of complexity in healthcare organisations, Kernick (2002), begins with the engaging observation that 'there is something not quite right with health service planning and delivery'. He refers to a series of studies which show that organisational change seems to have little impact on service provision, research has little influence on policy, many technical solutions developed by health economists have little effect at the front line of care, and that there is a persisting discrepancy between the impressive corporate images managers present (and presumably believe) and the reality of the experience of patients and staff. To this may be added problems of staff recruitment and retention, the common wish for early retirement – all this particularly among doctors, nurses and social workers, high levels of patient dissatisfaction with services, and high levels of litigation, staff sickness, absenteeism and suspension. All of which is extraordinarily costly, and not only in financial terms.

Kernick reviews the kinds of attempts made thus far to resolve such impediments to good service, which he identifies as managerial, hierarchical command and control; reliance on market forces with a division between providers and purchasers; and attempts to combine the two – a kind of 'third way' – with some kind of a balance being sought between central management and local autonomy. All of these, however, fall down because they are attempts to be scientific (in the way inadequate science was identified on page 24 *et seq*) in dealing with complex systems which are in fact beyond that kind of science. Kernick (2002) refers to these flawed attempts as the 'machine model', and one thinks of the steam engine trundling about and coming to a halt until Clark Maxwell taught its designers something about systems theory, as mentioned on page 34. Kernick's suggestions about dealing with complexity come down appropriately to a handful of simple-seeming questions about it:

- What does happen?
- What will happen?
- What would we like to happen?
- How can we make it happen?

All consistent, I think, with the question suggested here earlier: 'what's wanted, what's needed and what's possible?'

What happens is a salutary guide to what individuals and groups actually do as opposed to what they say, believe or are told they do. If facing the discrepancies revealed causes feelings of depression, we have seen (page 45) that depression, consequent on what psychoanalysts call reality-testing, *can* represent the beginning of change and creativity. What happens is also about aims which may be external to the group, and over which the group may have little or no control. Earlier I referred to the consultant's assumption of good intent. Thinking the best of the group, with its implications of being non-judgemental and morally neutral, may be important for the group's dynamic functioning and for the process of systems consultation, but as already said the consultant's personal values must be reflected in what he or she takes on in the first place. The consultant's job, once engaged in the work, is to help the institution operate. A consultant may not wish to help certain kinds of institution or team operate more effectively, and while it is not difficult to think up obvious examples (for example, prisons for political dissidents) there are many more subtle examples of settings where consultants may become less sure how their own values match those of the organisation.

The consultant should be able to handle very obvious dilemmas; it is the less obvious ones that may be more troubling, for the consultees even more than for the consultant. This is discussed further on page 66 *et seq*.

What will happen, for me, matches both exploration of fears, fantasy and wishes ('what's wanted?') and the realistic exploration of options ('what's needed').

What we would like to happen involves choice and decision making, which can be a good deal more difficult than the intelligent exploring of possibilities. It also represents a move from everyone democratically voicing their views to deciding how to make a decision, which invokes all the entrenched areas of authority and responsibility mentioned on page 51. To ask the innocent-seeming question 'How does this team usually make decisions?' can be an absolute spanner in the works, a real stopper, and should be used with care, but may be useful nonetheless.

Getting to *how can we make it happen*, if not easier, is at least likely to feel like a positive step, once decisions have been safely made, and may involve more readily handled matters such as those to do with the wider organisation, budgeting, planning and so on. However, while this stage of operational planning may afford some relief from contemplating feelings and the effects of feelings, and generate feelings of action and euphoria, there can be disappointments too.

The group consensus (to work out a decision, or to accept someone's individual decision) may not hold up once the external institutional difficulties are faced; compromises, back-tracking and other turbulence arises, and the paranoid ('it's all their fault', or power) and depressive ('it's our own fault', or weakness) cycle starts whirring again.

There can be great feelings of optimism when consultant and consultees meet for the first time; everything seems possible. Even the sceptics attend politely. However, it is wise to plan for regular review meetings specifically to assess progress, the basic agenda being what's working and what isn't working. This should include reflecting about the process of consultation itself: checking the machinery.

Institutions, even modest-seeming ones, are rock solid. That's how we like them. We also like seeing them change. This can be like carving in a stone composed of soft bits, brittle bits and areas like adamant. Mixed feelings, apprehension, depression, paranoia, anger all come into it, along with all the other myriad complexities of living systems.

Why it will all get worse

Well, it might not. The human race has an impressive record for muddling through the disasters it creates, though at huge cost, and I think it is quite feasible that in a hundred years from now a disaster-ridden, muddling-through world will be providing reasonable health services, especially for the children and grandchildren of the kind of people likely to read books like this. Probably healthcare will be increasingly impressive in many technical areas, and more or less deteriorating in provision for the chronic and intractable conditions, especially those of advanced age, and where it attempts to deal with the demand posed by victims of particular kinds of lifestyle, or people who feel victimised by life in general. I am not the first to be convinced that a large and growing sector will be those who are hopeful, or desperate, that science, via medicine, will fill the gap left by magic and religion – to make better the vicissitudes of life.

For all this, the poorer and technically less developed countries will probably want healthcare services just like ours. We will no doubt continue to have technical advance and popular demand haring into the future in a crazy game of leapfrog, while the deprived, wanting to emulate the high-tech West, will quite likely find themselves adding to their own problems those we have on our own lengthening healthcare agenda. However, being first in the race, we will no doubt continue to take their doctors and nurses to service our own insatiable demand. If we offer them teaching too, will it be useful back home? It is true that many non-Western countries have first-rate services. But many are based on a thriving private sector or the occasional centre of excellence; and more important, many have not yet begun to 'medicalise' an ever-wider range of problems in living in the way we have.

The core problem is of chaos arising out of complexity – a runaway and entirely open system. In essence, it is the problem of escalating demand for healthcare responses to conditions which are undefined and potentially unlimited. It is undefined and unlimited as far as the general public is concerned, as far as its ethical and legal advisers are concerned, as far as policy makers are concerned. It is undefined and unlimited as far as medical research is concerned, too; who, after all, would call a halt to any aspect of scientific progress? Thus there is an enormous and ever-expanding demand for an unspecified, fuzzy notion of what healthcare should take under its wings.

To list some of the factors enmeshed in this highly active other side of medicine:

1 Scientific research and other forms of enquiry will continue to plough ahead seeking new solutions to old problems, and identifying new problems needing solutions.

2 This, plus research and development, plus full implementation fast, will be backed to the hilt by just about everyone. There is a fine democracy in this, and of course votes too: everyone can pile into the queue with *their* needs as long as I can with mine.

3 There will be a sustained and justifiable expectation that one's individual problems will be dealt with promptly, without being held back by punishing waiting lists; and that once seen, sufficient time will be provided for proper assessment, treatment and follow-up. The economic requirements of providing adequate time for just three groups, for example – general practitioners' patients, people with emotional and psychiatric problems, and the unwell elderly – would mean an increase in expenditure, on average, of a factor of perhaps three or four *at the least*; that is, 300 or 400 per cent. However, that is only my guess, so no cause for alarm.

4 More and different conditions will come to light, identified by doctors, scientists, the general public and through the broadcasting and publishing media and the Internet. A substantial proportion of these

new problems will represent a kind of constant fallout from supposedly flawed diagnosis and treatment methods, many more from expectations of a better quality of life (e.g. in terms of mobility, longevity, brain function, confidence, appearance, behaviour, etc.), many from sources and forms of distress and frustration yet to be invented, and many resulting from 'lifestyle' (if it's the patient's fault) or social causes (if it's someone else's fault).

5　However, there is no evidence that any part of the policy-making spectrum, left, right or centre, democratic or authoritarian, could make a significant difference to this.

6　The proportion of the population living longer and with various degrees of managed disorder and disability will outpace the number of health-care practitioners young enough to train and work with them.

7　The ambivalent esteem in which healthcare workers and their colleagues are held – a mixture of high expectation and keen scepticism – will continue to challenge their authority, while piling on responsibilities. This source of demoralisation will add to the problems of lack of staff, particularly adequately trained staff. Problems in recruitment and retention of staff, premature retirement, suspensions, enquiries and litigation will grow. For who will call a halt?

8　There will be ever-increasing concern about the fitness and ability of healthcare staff, with their hurried training (training which as I hope this book shows, frequently misses the point), inadequate support and supervision, and their high turnover and high sickness rates. Increasing 'targets' set by desperate managers and politicians, trying to rationalise the irrational with increasing audit and revalidation, will add to the pressure. This system will become superheated as the necessary body of 'knowledge' expands, and more personnel have to audit, update and retrain, and to organise audit, updating and retraining. This particular system will probably be first in the race to critical mass and meltdown, those on the waiting lists being too unwell and apprehensive about hanging onto their place in the queue to riot.

9　Controversy among experts (and all the other commentators, which includes anyone with access to the Internet) will continue – about diagnosis, about general approaches and methods, about specific treatments.

10　Prevention will have to lag behind for lack of funding, lack of personnel and lack of a consensus about what is good for you.

11　The systems by which our healthcare services *do* manage to muddle along are themselves highly unstable. First, there is an astonishing tolerance of waiting lists, including long, long waits in Accident and Emergency Departments, and of avoidable mistakes; second, there is an absolutely enormous reliance on alternative and complementary therapies and on counselling services. Many are only doubtfully validated and regulated at present, although the validators and regulators are circling. 'Alternative' medicine carries a huge and growing load, but in general is treated by the 'mainstream' with suspicion. Do we know how much is useful?

12 An enormous weight of healthcare problems is born by social and care agencies and by charities and self-help groups, mostly, in various ways, struggling, and many (particularly the social and care services) vulnerable. This is particularly true as various versions of 'care in the community' are attempted.

13 While there tends to be universal controversy, scepticism, denial and deception about practically every facet and philosophy of politics and policy-making, there seems to be unanimity about one thing: Healthcare is Good. It is the new saintliness. If a problem can be medicalised, overtly or by stealth (e.g. by getting someone else to be 'doctor' and pretending that the medical model isn't being used – *see* page 151) it will generally receive popular support. If criminals can't simply be locked up at least they can be 'treated' as 'suffering from personality disorder', perhaps in advance. Such problems are then placed in a convenient category where doctors, therapists and scientists are doing the best they can with limited resources; and of course, here too, 'further research' is always in the pipeline.

14 I think it is true to say that as healthcare workers and patients we are not well equipped for the new questions being posed for healthcare as technical possibilities, general public and political expectations and the moral and ethical questions surrounding them burgeon. We are not all moral philosophers and up to date in everything. Issues involving genetics, contraception, abortion, euthanasia, 'living wills', compulsory treatment, the right *not* to treat, dangerousness, the medicalisation of a whole range of misbehaviour, and medical opinion expected to have 'scientific' answers to questions about dangerousness or what's best for a child and a family, could exercise a gathering of judges, philosophers and medical experts for ever; yet often such decisions have to be made urgently, and on the spot, by relatively inexperienced people, and sometimes with the pressure to decide coming from a range of strongly held and different opinions. And it is important to remember that it is not only the properly informed consent of the patient that is important here; the consent of the healthcare worker is a factor too.

These are some of the reasons why healthcare is complicated and getting more complicated, its common denominator being what Eisenberg (1975) described as the need to act amidst ambiguity. The *general* answer to some of this – the specifics are necessarily more complex – is a kind of mature negotiation which allows for the authority and wishes of the patient, the authority and wishes of the doctor, and mutual acceptance that options are vast and some decisions potentially very difficult. Systems consultation goes a long way towards achieving this kind of dialogue; patients as well as workers in the health fields might want to practice it.

CHAPTER 5

Theory to practice: principles, guidelines and some rules

- The story so far: a summary.
- Systems consultation as learning and teaching.
- Systems consultation as enquiry and research.
- Systems consultation as description.
- Consultation: practicalities, guidelines, hazards.

The story so far (continued)

Systems consultation has been described thus far as a method of joint enquiry whose particular style could help clarify complex and ambiguous issues in the healthcare field and assist decision making. It was presented as an approach which has, historically, grown out of more focused clinical forms of enquiry, so that we are left with two complementary procedures: traditional clinical consultation, which is suited to traditional concepts of medical problems, and systems consultation, which is suited to the wider, more complex systems which also affect clinical work, and which I have identified as the 'other' side of medical care. In the last chapter I suggested that it is this 'other' side which has been adding very substantially to the problems of providing healthcare, something which is likely to increase considerably over the coming years.

In this chapter we will stay with the basics of systems consultation and look at some of the guidelines and practicalities of undertaking it. In the subsequent four chapters we will look at different ways of using it, still with the purpose in mind of trying to bring clarity and focus to that which is ambiguous and diffuse in the delivery of medicine and healthcare.

One chapter – Chapter 8 – will consider the usefulness of using clinical consultation and systems consultation together as a kind of dual operating system, representing a widening of skills which could benefit everyone involved in clinical work. In Chapter 10 we will take the argument a step further, and suggest that the systemic consultative style which was originally designed for collaboration between professional specialists may be useful for work with another kind of expert: the patient.

'The joint exploration of what is wanted, what is needed and what is possible': a deconstruction

- **Joint**: Those needed to make a decision or choice. The information each brings to the consultation, and their respective expectations and roles, are different; their discussion is on an equal basis.
- **What is wanted**: An amalgam of wishes, hopes, expectations, anticipations and fears, based on information of variable validity and reliability, and motivated by both rational and emotional influences.
- **What is needed**: This represents a first stage of negotiation; it is a kind of shared assessment, with the healthcare worker contributing his or her special knowledge and experience, and the other, whether professional or patient, theirs.
- **What is possible**: This is what they discover: the options available, their relative merits, what each side feels about them, priorities, and the process of making a decision.

The learning principle

Any impression that the whole point of systems consultation is primarily as a polite exercise in democracy is wrong. Conceivably its principles might provide a viable framework for real, as opposed to pretend, democracy, but that is a question for political philosophers.

The central tenet of the kind of consultation described here is that it is a learning and teaching exercise in a world where choices have to be made but no one has all the answers. In this sense it is a contribution, and I think could be a major one, to the principle of 'lifelong learning' – where everyone, without exception, has to keep up with different and changing values as well as advances and opinions in one's own specialist field.

After a worthwhile exercise in consultation the consultee ought to know more than he or she realised before about:

- the matter which was the focus of consultation
- old and new information relevant to this focus
- what he or she can do about it
- what it is reasonable to expect colleagues to contribute
- what should be expected from the work setting in general

- how consultation works
- how he or she works
- how to manage equivalent situations next time.

Clearly this is a long way from simply being told 'how to do it', and a world away from someone doing it for you.

What is just as important is that *the consultant learns too*, in each of the above areas.

Consultation as research

Consultation brings together three areas which unfortunately tend to drift apart: clinical practice, learning and research. This is partly because people tend to be appointed primarily as teachers, researchers or clinicians and then get increasingly busy with their personal or institutional priorities, emphasising one of these at the expense of the others (incidentally, an interesting focus for consultation). All three areas lose from this. As Taylor (1986) has pointed out, not all research has to be 'big science', though its increasing volume and prestige has made it seem like that; rather, systematic enquiry is integral to both learning and clinical practice.

There are many ways of adding research to clinical work, but even a small-scale study or single case report has its own discipline in terms of methodology and the time it needs. The consultative approach isn't a substitute for this, but it does foster real curiosity about the core clinical problem and the very much wider context clinical problems occur in. This is good for the particular matter in hand, and as we have seen, for the further education of both consultant and consultee. However, it is also good for the way professions work, replacing the processing of patients with a spirit of enquiry which could even be professionally and personally refreshing, perhaps reminding us of why we entered our field of work in the first place. Further, the wide net that systems consultation casts makes it possible to generate new and unusual hypotheses for formal research projects.

Consultation as description

The work is *descriptive*, not diagnostic or prescriptive. Description is an account – a narrative – of what is happening, not an interpretation or diag-nosis of what is happening. The motivation of the people involved (including the consultee) is not part of the discussion; however, the conse-quences are. Dealing with the implications and results of personal issues indirectly, insofar as it affects work, is part of the skill of the work. This is described in several examples in the next few chapters; for example, should a consultee explain difficulties in the job because of 'feeling depressed lately', the consultative work does not shift perspective and become clinical, but helps the consultee think through how his depressed feelings relate to and affect the work and what he thinks he should do about it. Similarly with a consultee/colleague with supposed emotional or personality problems: the consultee is not encouraged to take on a therapeutic and diagnostic role towards them, but to consider what the options are if their job is to be done properly (*see* Examples 6, 7 and 8).

In relation to professional skills, suppose a consultee sees, as a result of consultation, that her client – for example, a child in a children's home – would benefit from regular counselling sessions. The consultation should explore how this suggestion will be taken further, how and by whom, and shouldn't in general change tack to helping the consultee provide counselling. I say 'in general' because systems consultation shouldn't be rigid; it would not be ruled out that the consultation session could look at how conversations with the child were going, at whether this indicated that something more systematic might help, whether the consultee had the experience and the role to provide it, and what supervision he or she might want. But the consultative session would not drop everything else and change direction in order to provide it.

Again, the same applies to teaching. A teacher (as consultee) might see that a systematic, behavioural approach to a child's problems may be worth trying, and the consultation session could explore how this could be provided; but it would not be for the consultation session to turn itself into a kind of short training course in behaviour therapy. However, this statement needs to be qualified. First, the consultant might be able and willing to describe what a behavioural approach would entail, and to see if it is needed and wanted; second, some psychologists specifically provide *behavioural consultation*, a category of consultative work in which the specifically agreed focus for work is to help teachers apply behavioural regimes (e.g. Conoley and Conoley 1982; Tattum 1986; Topping 1986).

In summary, to keep systems consultation on target, the focus is to demonstrate what's happening and what the consultee wants and then plans to do about it; not to do it. But this does not preclude the consultant, by virtue of his or her particular background, suggesting things to look for that the consultee might not have thought of, or approaches that the consultee seems not to know about.

How to proceed when asked to provide consultation

This outline assumes an invitation to provide systems consultation to a group, with the focus primarily on how the consultees work or on developing their skills.

First contact

First, find out what is wanted. Just because 'consultation' has been asked for doesn't mean that is what is wanted. It cannot be overemphasised that you may well be asked for consultation when supervision is wanted, or vice versa. Second, find out who wants it. The consultee or consultees must be in a position to put into practice whatever emerges from consultation.

Example 1: the authority of the consultee

A staff nurse asks a specialist registrar if she could provide consultative sessions to the nurses on an intensive care unit for children, to help them reflect about how they handle parents' feelings. It seems a good idea. The staff nurse has discussed it with the unit's senior nurse over coffee, and with one of the unit's consultant paediatricians, and both thought it an excellent and 'supportive' idea. However, the senior nurse hadn't considered that what the nursing group learned from the sessions might well change several details of how they work, and would have implications for the administration of the unit. Also, the other consultant paediatricians with beds on the unit didn't know about the scheme, which would affect how their patients were handled.

Comments

Consultation isn't merely 'supportive', except as a helpful side effect; it generates new ideas, some of them worth implementing, and more people would have needed to know about the nurse's request than two or three people who thought (correctly) that it was a good idea. Given an invitation like this you could suggest that the staff nurse meets the paediatricians and senior nurse and talks through with them the idea; you could suggest inviting yourself along for what is in effect a preliminary ('pre-consultation') consultation; or you could suggest a one-off exploratory teaching session with the nursing group – with the agreement and ideally the presence of the nurse in charge – to see what comes up and where, if anywhere, they want to take the idea next; for example, to any nursing or unit planning meeting. This may sound overcautious and fussy, but, first, you do need eyes in the back of your head when agreeing to this kind of move; and second, it is a matter of teasing out the complex lines of authority and accountability in which the consultees-to-be are enmeshed, not just to avoid embarrassment (though this is useful) but to respect the existing lines of decision making because these are what the consultees will have to use to take any further action.

Second contact

Mentioned for completeness; it may for example be the 'pre-consultation consultation', when as consultant-to-be you discuss with the consultees-to-be who would like you to do what, and who else should be involved.

Formalities

Do *you* need anyone's permission to use your time in this way? When and where are you going to meet? Will it be a single meeting, or a series? Will those who are interested always be able to attend? (Particularly for people on rotas, for example nursing and care staff.) If not, will a changing group population work? Depending on whether organisational boundaries are being crossed, will you or your department be paid for your sessions? Do you know what the charge should be, if payment is to be made? Are you happy with an informal agreement, or should someone write to confirm it? In some cases, for example if a medium- to long-term number of sessions are needed, a formal agreement or contract might be needed.

Are you going to keep notes? And the question of confidentiality

You should keep notes, even if they are minimal, for example keeping a 'diary' of date, who was present and the matter discussed. Confidentiality is important. You can try not to identify patients or clients or other people outside the group, but names do slip out, and patients attending a particular department, clinic or practice different to your own will not expect their names to be recorded in the notes of your own workplace. If you follow the principles suggested here for consultation, remember that you are helping your consultee, in privacy and confidentiality, not the person the consultee is talking about; if your consultee wants to talk about X or Y being an alcoholic or otherwise unfit for their work, it is the *consultee's* work problem you are discussing, not X's or Y's supposed clinical state. I believe this understanding, if adhered to, supports the integrity of this sort of work, but vigilance and respect for X's or Y's privacy and confidentiality (not quite the same thing) are essential, and my own view is that their identities should not emerge in the consultative meeting, still less be recorded. It may be that difficult issues of confidentiality may arise in group consultation, and that you may already have decided that for reasons of practicality the group will be 'open', with a shifting membership; and that the organisation to whom you are consulting itself has staff, perhaps from agencies, who come and go. All these factors can present confidentiality problems.

There are wider issues, also, than those concerning individuals. In cross-agency work (for example, meeting nurses from a number of practices, or counsellors with a number of clinical attachments) people might allege things about identifiable units or organisations which they would hesitate to say about individual people.

These are all difficult areas for systems consultation. The requirement that the consultee be regarded as a competent professional, and treated as a peer, applies also to how seriously they take the question of confidentiality.

There may be times, perhaps when trying to help a floundering and even chaotic organisation, for example an overstretched children's home with serious shortcomings attributed to individuals, when the consultant might be of best service by limiting what is discussed in an open group, and consulting with the consultees about how else their concern may be handled; for example administratively, if necessary, rather than through continuing consultation (*see* also Example 8).

The process of consultation

The following list represent the kinds of stages the consultation process proceeds through, possibly in something like this order, though the work will develop a dynamism of its own, with steps on the following agenda being returned to and reworked from time to time. This is a natural process – in ordinary situations people get to know each other and work on things in similarly roundabout and spiralling ways. The examples in the next few chapters contain examples of some of the key steps and developments.

- Introducing yourself and each other. A brief and informal statement about who you are, how you got to be there and why you understand you're there is a helpful courtesy. But *brief*. An apprehensive group or individual might well allow you to turn this into a short lecture if you aren't careful.
- Asking people to describe what they do – again, briefly, and initiating a discussion about the 'agenda': what you understand the meeting is for, and what the consultees think. I do not recommend the 'silent group' start, with group tension mounting until someone 'breaks' or thinks up something to say. This is common in group psychotherapy where it may serve particular purposes (e.g. to raise emotional arousal) and is sometimes encouraged by people doing consultative work whose hearts are in psychotherapy (*see* pages 18, 103–4). However, there may be times for reflective quiet, particularly when a group has got to know each other; and it is also important that individuals do not dominate the group, or try to avoid silence, by chattering. It is a consultative skill – introduced by the consultant, learned by the consultees – to get the

balance right between useless silence and useless noise. If in doubt: consult the consultees, of course.

The consultant should hold in his or her head a kind of rolling agenda: all sorts of important matters may be mentioned mildly, shyly, inconsequentially or in fairly inarticulate ways. This is precisely *because* the 'institution' (i.e. the group, or the work setting) will have its own narrative or language to keep it going in a particular direction (including round and round in circles) and the consultative group may be the first and only occasion to attempt a different kind of conversation. Not knowing what's going on, admitting bafflement about who in the institution does what and why, not knowing the extent of one's own role and skills in relation to others, not knowing how to put it or how to explain – all this is the material that matters, and if the consultation is going well it may come too thick and fast to attend to all at once. The consultant should be custodian, archivist and, in due course – jointly with the consultees – editor of this important 'cutting-room floor' data.

I would confirm when the meeting is to end, as part of the introduction, and remind everyone about confidentiality.

- There follows the circular process of getting to know (in order to trust) each other, getting to know about the work setting (often an eye-opener for the consultees who work there, as well as for the visiting consultant) and clarifying the task for consultation. In this process there should develop what Campbell calls the process of creating a climate for working together (Campbell, 1999) and which I would equate with Winnicott's facilitating environment, and with Bowlby's safe base from which risk-laden exploration becomes possible (Bowlby 1969; Winnicott 1972; and pages 46–7).

One of the items on the consultant's agenda is for the issues behind the issues. The overt task for consultation is likely to be resting on other, more fundamental matters; e.g. unhappiness about how a particular way of working is developing may be a fig leaf for the more troubling issue of disquiet about how decisions are made in the organisation, and by whom. It is not for the consultant to jump in with an interpretation about this though he or she is bound to sometimes make tentative assumption which may or may not be valid. But if such subterranean matters seem to be producing tremors again and again, the consultant should find ways of making it alright for the group to explore them. If they don't want to, or can't, it may have to wait until they do, and can.

- As problems become clarified, they should (if the consultation has been clearing the undergrowth) look unmanageable, chaotic and perhaps a bit crazy. Organisations are like that. But even the most complex muddles can be organised into manageable pieces and prioritised. 'Bits' can be distributed chronologically – one thing at a time – or to different consultees. At this point one may mention changing tack into one of a number of 'action' or creative techniques which are discussed later, for example using subgroups to meet about one aspect of a problem and reporting back, or using sculpting or art techniques, or simply drawing things up on a flip chart or white board. These techniques are described in Examples 14–17. Such primarily non-verbal strategies have the advantage of finding ways to describe problems and solutions outside the official, correct language and formulae of the organisation.

Changing gear to such alternative strategies requires explanation – perhaps along the above lines – and the consultees' agreement. Consultation is about trying to clarify, and helping the consultees to find comfortable ways of working; not trying to mystify, still less trying to show what a magician the consultant is.

- History is important – not a clinical-type history but the narratives, official and unofficial, so far; of the organisation, of the people working there, of the emergence of assorted problems and solutions, including the story of what used to happen, how some solutions have worked or half-worked. Abandoned part-solutions are a rich source of possibilities that could work next time. All this is likely to be part fact, part myth, part fiction, part real and part imagined biography.

- By the same token reflection about how the future, even as fantasy, certainly as wishful thinking, can be helpful, because it is likely to be a repository of the seeds of useful and useable ideas; and energising and optimistic too. Meanwhile the consultant will be aware of the mood of the group – thus moving from describing supposedly insoluble problems to fantasising about possible futures can represent a shift from depression to a better mood. Experienced consultants and consultees become able to comment lightly on this without heavy-handed interpretations; stating – merely reflecting – e.g. how the mood of the group seems to provide feedback and help achieve homeostatic balance between pessimism and optimism or between cognitive (intellectual) and emotional activity. It is another example of the consultant having confidence in the group's capacity, away from the pressures, distractions and business of the job, for imaginative, creative appraisal and self-appraisal – comparable, I think, to Sluzki's (1999) notion of assuming good intent.

- On page 48 I referred to 'reversion to what used to work' as an explanation of behaviour within the attachment model of human functioning, and which could apply to either disturbed or to normal behaviour: nature doesn't comment on the difference. Thus the normal kind of excited anticipation or apprehension that might precede, say, theatrical or sporting performance, might owe something to earlier childlike ways of carrying on without being in the slightest way abnormal; nor, necessarily, are people's individual ways of coping with it. At this normal level, a first consultative meeting might generate varying degrees of apprehension, and some members adopt the kind of strategies they ordinarily find familiar and supportive. Thus, someone part-experienced in psychotherapy or counselling might be moved to comment on their or the groups's feelings, someone else come armed with a clipboard and pen or memo pad, and a senior person might feel obliged to make a short, or even extended, explanatory speech. I would let such things pass unless or until such strategies get in the way of other people's contributions, though I would discourage private note-taking at the time if the other consultees agreed it was inappropriate.

But *why* might it be inappropriate? Because the group is essentially experimental; it is being encouraged to play with ideas; it should not be like an administrative, decision-making meeting; the work of the group is work in progress; as said earlier, ideas which emerge are for the others present to try on for size, if they wish, or to stimulate their own ideas; action and decisions are for later, and these may be personal decisions or matters put on the agenda of a decision-making meeting. The only intellectual case for taking notes during the meeting would be if the processes of the meeting were being researched in some way, which would need explanation and agreement. What private notes people keep for themselves, afterwards, is a private matter, and I would anticipate this possibility by mentioning this too in the context of confidentiality

Ending meetings

This is handled by some consultants in the style of some psychotherapists: as the clock ticks to the end of whatever time has been agreed (which it should be), if someone is in mid-flow many consultants would start to gather themselves together to leave. There may or may not be a polite show of fast-diminishing interest, the message being that what is being said must wait for next time, with the admonitory subtext that it should have been brought up earlier. My own view is that – as well as the room having a reliable clock – the consultant should draw the group's attention to the fact when the last few minutes are approaching. And end on time.

   Ending a series of meetings requires anticipation and allowance for all kinds of feelings about the series. It is helpful to discuss what to 'take home', in the sense of back to work, and how, and to acknowledge in this respect how different from the consultative meetings 'back home' is likely to be.

Summary: some rules for systems consultation

1 The consultant's job is to help the consultees do theirs, not to do it for them (*see* Example 3).
2 Identifying a need for consultation about a problem or issue is something for the consultees to decide; and describing it and possible

solutions should be in the consultees' terms, words and ways of working, not in those of the background discipline of the consultant (*see* Example 2).

3 The common language of consultation for consultant and consultees to use as a *lingua franca* should be plain English (or, of course, whatever the prevailing demotic language happens to be).

4 The consultee's work status, training, responsibility and authority need to be broadly commensurate with the problem or issue being discussed. This rule, a particularly important one, may be stated as *going in at the right level* (*see* Example 1).

5 Since Rule 4 cannot always be precisely defined, especially in complex work systems, the consultant should be alert to that which is usefully discussible within the consultation (i.e. what the consultees can decide about and act on for themselves), and that which they would be better advised to 'distil out' of the consultation session into whatever administrative meetings or line management machinery exist in their work; or to set up such machinery if none suitable exists (*see* Examples 6 and 8).

6 The process of consultation can be a little like psychotherapy in some respects, but is significantly different, particularly in being concerned with what happens, not why, and in being focused on various outcomes in terms of people's jobs (*see* Example 7).

7 Consultation may overlap with supervision in training, but should not be confused with hierarchical, line-management supervision, which would be seriously misleading and can be potentially disastrous.

8 Consultation is like some forms of teaching, but whether the consultation is meeting primarily for problem-handling or primarily as a training exercise should be clear to consultant and consultees (*see* Example 9).

9 All this should form the basis of an agreement with the consultees and their employers, circumstances dictating whether this dual contract can be informal or in writing (*see* Example 10).

10 Consultative work should be pragmatic and helpful. The rules can be adapted to the matter in hand *in consultation with the consultees* if there is a good reason to do so and if the principles of the first nine rules are understood. When in doubt or when reviewing anything at all consult the consultees (*see* Example 11).

Summary of pitfalls to avoid

- Going in at the wrong level of authority, information and responsibility. The *possession on the part of the consultee of enough information about a problem and its setting to get started* is essential.
- Thinking you are providing consultation when the consultees and/or

their employers (and thus, often, your employer) believe you to be providing hierarchical, line-management supervision.

- Thinking you are providing consultation when the consultees and/or their employers think you are providing psychotherapy, counselling or 'support'.
- Being clinical: working with your own skills 'through' the consultee, for example getting them to take a medical history by proxy.
- Acting as an advocate or activist: many issues are political in terms of power structures, economics and fairness in the organisation, and while relevant ones will properly become clarified in consultation it is not for the consultant to prompt the consultees to particular courses of action. Like everything else, motivation and action is up to them.
- Not being vigilant about confidentiality because the sessions are not clinical.

CHAPTER 6

Consultation with working groups and organisations

> *Examples*:
> - Care skills in a residential setting.
> - Psychiatry in the classroom.
> - Speaking the same language.
> - Precision about participants.
> - The agenda – and other agendas.
> - Consultation, not therapy.
> - Consultation, not management.
> - Work focus *vs* training focus.
> - Contracts, confidentiality, privacy.
> - The rules, and when to bend them.

Introduction

I have differentiated between working groups and organisations in the title because sometimes the working group *is* the whole organisation, e.g. a clinic or practice team, and sometimes it is a team or unit within it.

As pointed out at the beginning of the previous chapter, we will use the fundamentals of inter-professional systems consultation for the time being in order to illustrate its essentials, although later in the book we will be seeing how these consultative strategies between professional workers can be adapted for direct work with our clients and patients.

The rest of this chapter uses examples of episodes in consultative work to illustrate some basic rules and guidelines. The examples are a reminder that systems consultation with an organisation may be on a single occasion, though further meetings with a slightly different agenda may be sought later. Alternatively, an organisation may request regular sessions with an outside consultant.

Example 2: the autonomy of the consultees

The Head of a residential school for children with special needs asks the school medical officer if she would take a staff group to help them review how they handle some of the physical, emotional and behavioural problems that arise there. The Head isn't happy with the way a number of things are being handled, for example children's idiosyncrasies, real and imagined, allergies, medication. There have also been a number of complaints from parents about how some of their worries and complaints have been responded to. The doctor, vaguely assuming an appreciative meeting with the staff, is taken aback when, after a few courtesies, a considerable amount of resentment starts coming through. The doctor was anticipating a useful discussion about parental anxieties about institutions, children's problems and medication and so on; instead the group comes alive and very heated on the question of how the staff feel unappreciated and constantly criticised. What the staff bring up *does* seem very important; it just wasn't expected, and when the doctor tries to raise the kinds of issues raised by the Head she is accused of just joining in with the general criticism of a staff group which is feeling overstretched and unappreciated. Reporting back to the Head (by then in receipt of a formal complaining letter about the group from a staff representative), the doctor finds the Head, too, floundering somewhat and rather worried about how to handle a rising tide of parental complaints and questions from social workers while the staff are becoming ever more thinly stretched and demoralised.

Comments

1   The doctor, innocently trying to help with what she thought would be a helpful and even pleasant seminar on working with children and parents, finds herself instead with an open can of worms. For the purposes of this example I will not attempt to go into the handling of all its ramifications; but it illustrates what Caplan (1970) called *mandated* consultation, and is quite a common error. Remember, the rule is the expectation that the staff seen in consultation – the consultees – should have the wish, the information and the status, i.e. the potential, to do something with whatever useful emerges from consultation. In mandated consultation A (the Head) asks B (the consultant) to please see C (the consultees) about something A thinks is amiss. The consultees, with heaven knows what expectations about the meeting (announced by memo from the Head: 'Dr B would like to meet the staff in Houses X and Y in the library at 6pm to discuss the handling of the children') have agendas of their own, mostly about feeling under siege.

2   Setting off on the right track would have required a first consultation with the Head, about the problems as he perceived them. It is possible

that one or two systems consultations focused on matters the Head was trying to sort out would have been all that was needed. Or, thinking of Example 6, it is conceivable that the consultation might have identified things to take to his own Governors, or to whatever meetings he held regularly with the staff. (And if there weren't any, this could raise the question whether such a meeting might be useful.)

3   A meeting between the Head and the staff, with someone not directly involved in the school's day-to-day running (possibly but not necessarily the doctor) acting as its facilitator could be a useful next step to see what kinds of things ought to be on the agenda for Head and staff to review.

4   Two things for example might emerge from a successful meeting between the Head and the staff. First, regular, non-crisis meetings between Head and staff about how things were going in the running of the school. Second, the staff might like to have some consultative – teaching meetings (Example 9) with the school doctor about the kinds of health and care problems and parental concerns that the care staff were regularly faced with.

5   Two kinds of consultative meetings could now replace the emotionally charged muddle of the first. The meeting between head and staff about the way the school is run brings together the people who would know the score about the problems that the staff and Head originally perceived separately; it would be important in a meeting like that for the consultant to acknowledge the respective authority and roles of those present, and within which each would be autonomous. The second meeting would be more like the teaching meeting the Head originally had in mind, but now with the staff wanting it to happen. School administration now firmly back on the Head's desk, this time with the staff working on it with him.

Example 3: the consultee's perspective as primary

Two child specialists are asked to help two schools with consultative meetings about problem behaviour among the pupils. Dr Y is a behavioural psychologist, and Dr Z a child psychiatrist with a special interest in family and group psychotherapy. Imagine an examination question: you are asked to compare and contrast the kinds of things Dr Y and Dr Z each expect to be discussing. Will Dr Y anticipate discussing the importance of identifying wanted and unwanted behaviour, and different ways of reinforcing one and discouraging the other? Will Dr Z, however, want to remind the teachers about the group dynamics of the classroom and the various ways that the dynamics of each child's family might enter the classroom?

The right answer (I would say) is that both Dr Y and Dr Z should be willing and able to suspend the application of their respective ways of thinking about children's problems, and instead be occupied with: what is this school like? What are the teachers and the children like? What kinds of problems are the teachers concerned about? How do they usually respond? What happens then? And above all, in what terms do they describe all this? Do Dr Y or Dr Z know what kinds of backgrounds the teachers have, and how much and what kind of teaching or experience each might have had on this subject? How will they find out? How does the classroom look through their (the teachers') eyes? How does the help available (e.g. from the school, but also from people like Dr Y or Dr Z) look like from their points of view? What do they hope for from the meeting?

Comments

1   That, I suggest, is the way to start. It does not preclude Dr Y or Dr Z bringing in their own perspectives if requested, or if it feels appropriate to do so, for example the consultant matching his or her narratives with that of the teachers, to see what kind of mix and match the teachers think will help them in their own work. Do not, however, underestimate how difficult it is for a highly trained specialist, or a highly trained generalist for that matter, to hold back, refrain from telling (or hinting at) what to do, and instead to simply observe what's going on and see how the consultees are trying to handle things using their own training and experience. Consultation is different: it is not like clinical work; although teaching and learning is reciprocal in consultation (*see* page 99 *et seq*), for the consultant the cycle starts with learning.

2   But shifting the goalposts is all right. *Anything* is all right if discussed and agreed between consultant and consultees. The teachers in one of the schools might request a teaching session and not consultation at all. They will need to sort out whether this would be a one-off didactic talk, or whether they are looking for a series of training sessions or even regular supervision in this aspect of their work. In which case would Dr Y mention Dr Z's kind of approach, and vice versa? Or the place of medication for some kinds of behavioural problems?

Example 4: plain English as the official language of consultation

I dislike jargon and am suspicious of most 'politically correct' forms of expression, and hope I haven't slipped too much into these here. However, what is technical language or shorthand to one person can be annoying and incomprehensible jargon to another. With all these styles people have their preferences and habits, avoiding some while taking others for granted in conversation. The problem is that many different disciplines meet in the health and care field and what is straightforward plain English to one person may sound like obscure or pretentious jargon (like 'psychobabble') to another. However, the point is not to encourage or ban particular forms of expression, but to take it for granted that not everyone will necessarily understand everyone else's usage, and full comprehension by all concerned is essential in consultative work. Earlier in the book I referred to administrative meetings being conducted in the modern Western equivalent of Mandarin Chinese, and with much the same purpose, that is the excluding, in-group confirming the language of the governing elite. I think its purpose is less to confuse the peasants than to remind them who's the boss, and that if you aspire to have your comments paid attention to, you must use the same dialect. It also makes the mundane sound conveniently profound to those who matter, and leaves the others in the dark. It should be part of the ethos of consultative work to invite consultant or consultees to explain, or translate, if what they have said isn't crystal clear to all.

My 'example' is actually composed of a number of experiences with interpreters, sometimes when working with a family, sometimes in a consultative work with staff groups and sometimes when teaching (Steinberg 2000d). The 'common sense' assumption might be that using an interpreter makes things more difficult. It certainly makes conversation slower. However, my impression is that with a good, painstaking interpreter, one who will carefully discuss (consult) with consultant, consultees (or patients or trainees) about whether the phrase chosen is the best one, the purpose and content of the conversation can actually become clearer and closer to intended meanings on all sides than had all participants been supposedly speaking the same language. The interpreter then becomes a participant in the consultation, with the communication of intended meaning being central to the task, not a mere peripheral aid or convenience. In fact the appearance of speaking the same language can make people think they understand each other when they don't. But perhaps this is the fundamental nature of the consultant's task: to interpret the narrative.

So this aspect of my account of consultation has gone full circle, from urging the use of plain English to saying 'be careful' because in some circumstances even plain English may not be all that it seems. Thus consultation is full of surprises, as it should be.

Example 5: having the necessary people present

Several senior and middle grade people in a clinical department think they should have a meeting to discuss recurring team problems, most of which centre on the senior consultant, a man whose retirement is not very far off: only about four years. He is the kind of person described in obituaries as one of the old school, the kind of character you don't see any more, 'capable of enormous kindness' but 'not someone who suffered fools gladly'.

He does things his own way, and doesn't fit in easily with team discussions and decisions or any of the usual channels. He is a workaholic, and on a more serious note is thought by the gossipers to be possibly an alcoholic, possibly depressed. He arrives late for conferences and ward rounds, but demands that everyone else should be on the spot on time, and the meetings overrun. Some brave souls eventually leave before the meeting's over, without complaint by the consultant, but the team's 'punishment' is that some decisions are made without the right people there, and others get vaguely postponed. Most people kind of like him, and are infuriated by him. The most sustainable and least embarrassing complaint that the team can agree on is to state as a general problem the fact that the department's timetable is proving hard to adhere to and that decisions get made informally without key people knowing. One of the senior nurses takes on the task of trying to coordinate a meeting at a time suitable for everyone. One of the specialist registrars is persuaded to have a word with the senior person about having a special meeting to discuss these matters, and is immensely heartened when the senior consultant says what an excellent idea it is; indeed he'd been thinking along just the same lines himself but wondering how to bring it up. It proves difficult to arrange a time that suits everyone, but some months after the idea first emerged the time, place and a tray of tea and biscuits are all set up, for the end of a busy day, of course. The key man is late, as usual; but more than late. Twenty minutes after the scheduled start the specialist registrar receives a call on his mobile phone to say that unfortunately the senior consultant is involved in a meeting on the other side of the city, and which has had to overrun. 'But you go ahead, and I'll be very happy to go along with anything you decide.'

Comments

1   Thus with one bound Dr X is free, and not for the first time. Indeed the politics of his career, both in broad perspective and in detail, is represented in the microcosm of this attempted meeting. He habitually controls his colleagues by finely tuned affability on the one hand and irascibility on the other, and at any given time his allies on any issue, great and small, outnumber those whom he is currently causing severe proctalgia. Determined informality and the avoidance of embarrassment are the twin pillars of his approach to his colleagues, and the meeting has been set up, and abandoned, on just these principles. The answer is to arrange a more formal meeting.

2   The most important matter – whether the man would be there – had been unwisely shunted to one side and left to wishful thinking. In fact the matter should have been central, and he and his secretary asked if they would set the meeting up, as it was crucial for the team's most authoritative figure to be present. The single item for the agenda could

have been stated at the same time, and quite directly without causing the much-feared embarrassment: that the way the department operated frequently required his presence, but fixing punctual and focused meetings which reached viable decisions had become impracticable. He was needed to help them sort it out. If the suggestion came back, probably through his secretary, that the others had his permission to sort it out, this should be politely but firmly refused. He was the important figure and they needed him to be there.

3   The powerful collusion to avoid an embarrassing scene was due, of course, to the fact that the issue had become highly personalised, with individuals feeling considerable anger and some apprehension, even vaguely contemplated fantasies about the consultant's health, and how on earth he might respond. However, the meeting is not 'about' the senior consultant; it is about the team's ability to hold punctual, reliable, predictable meetings with a reasonable agenda and the right people present to make sustainable decisions. This is not a ploy, but true: however, it is in the nature of manipulative behaviour that attempts to be straight feel emotive and manipulative. If he turns out to be quite unable or unwilling to meet his colleagues predictably when his presence and attention is needed to discuss cases and make decisions, then this has the makings of a rather serious issue, and might need to be on the agenda of more formal meetings still (as discussed in different circumstances in Examples 6 and 8).

4   Depending on how seriously the proposal for a meeting is taken, it might well need to be notified to all concerned in writing, with definite starting and ending times, and promptness being stressed. For anyone unable to attend, the note would have indicated that the meeting would need to be rescheduled. Persistence and clarity of focus are likely to be needed, not anger, exasperation or nagging.

5   It may seem that only one matter among many will be discussed, but if it is dealt with properly other matters will fall into line, just as – in the department's prevailing management style – matters have so far fallen out of line. For example: if the clinical meetings happened properly, then the many informal, chaotic discussions and proposals in corridors, the car park (engine running) or over the phone that thus far patched up the disorganised meetings would become redundant. They would instead be referred back to whichever was the proper meeting. *This* might produce a major or minor explosion, but that would be another matter. Thus, pulling one thing into line, if accurately identified as a problem and properly dealt with, pulls other things back into line too. All this may sound unduly pedantic and controlling, but that is how delinquency is dealt with. Informality is preferable, as long as it works both ways.

6   But prevention is better than cure. One answer, as suggested on page

86, is for any team which is at all elaborate and complex to have three sorts of meetings: clinical conferences, which they would have in any case; administrative, decision-making meetings at whatever intervals are necessary; and, from time to time, a non-clinical, non-administrative meeting to discuss feelings and the 'fallout' from day-to-day work in terms of what's going well and what needs to be improved: *not* in terms of personalities or values, but in terms of working relationships, and with the focus on the work. As said earlier, people and their working relationships are the key tools for healthcare work, and should be kept in good order.

Example 6: identifying items for other kinds of agendas

A consultant meets a group of college counsellors regularly to discuss their work with their students. One counsellor is in an uncharacteristic state of anxiety about an unhappy young man who is demanding more and more of her time, and whose work and social life is deteriorating, with increasing alienation from his parents and friends. The counsellor fears something dreadful will happen – suspension from the college, even self-injury or suicide. She finds it hard to assess his degree of depression, having observed him looking quite cheerful among his peers, but whenever she sees him he seems distressed and hopeless. She has floated the idea of a psychiatric opinion, which the student regarded as the counsellor rejecting him, indeed treating the idea as deliberate referral to a service that would be unhelpful if not punitive. When the group looks at the wider system in which student and counsellor are enmeshed, two things are volunteered. First, her marriage is going through a rocky period, and one of the many causes of distress is that the student reminds her of the present unhappiness and insecurity of her own son, the only child – also a student – still living at home. Second, the consultant asks the counsellor about something she already appreciates, that therapeutic work stirs up the therapist's feelings too, and these can get in the way of the work, and asks what supervision she receives. The answer is none; it's just not been allowed for, neither within the college nor in her own wider professional arrangements. She knows of the local branch of an organisation that provides systematic supervision for counsellors but hasn't seen the need for it, nor is sure she can find the time to go. The other consultees, several of whom do have regular supervision, say how helpful it is; and after a time the consultee says she does realise that, but is reluctant to take time away from home in the evening just when her son needs her most, seeing supervision sessions as a kind of luxury indulgence, one that – she thinks – her husband could add to his list of resentments. She also feels – quite irrationally, she herself says that with her current domestic and emotional problems she might somehow lose control in the challenging and emotive atmosphere she imagined goes with formal supervision sessions. Talking this through in the group she decides to go for supervision after all; and, with her husband, to think about marital counselling. Simply to have made two personal decisions helps her get her client's problems into a better perspective, and she begins to feel better about her work with him even before following up the two steps she proposed.

Another college counsellor puzzled the group a little because although clearly highly competent in her work, there seemed to be with one student a mystery impediment in the way. Then the counsellor described the awkwardness of her part-time office, which amounted to a very exposed if relatively soundproof glass-walled corner of a huge office floor. She and her clients had two chairs and a coffee table in front of the desk of the secretary who used the office the rest of the time. The phone would ring briefly from time to time before an inaudible message-system picked up the call; and staff approaching the huge windows, seeing counselling going on, would discreetly veer away. So that was all right.

The consultation group asked if a counselling situation like that could be tolerated. From this it emerged that the arrangement was an improvement on what had prevailed before, when the counsellor had operated in a screened-off area of a large engineering workshop area; and from this it was a short step into the history of the job, which had started out as a kind of vocational counselling-cum-first-aid nurse (the students would occasionally hurt themselves mildly while working the machinery). The consultee had got the job because it had been recognised that personal counselling was what the present generation of students, and staff, were looking for; but the facilities had stayed much the same, including the first-aid box with which she was provided. The group became interested in her job description, which turned out to be the original one of a kind of counselling nurse; and the consultee decided to go and see the vice principal about it. He turned out to be only too pleased to organise a more appropriate contract for her, one that fitted what she actually did, instead of what people 25 years before had wanted, and – once the problem was put before him – could see that she had to have a more appropriate office too.

Comments

1   Both examples illustrate the importance of wide-ranging detective work into questions about the tools needed for the job, and what it took to obtain them and keep them in good shape. In the first case the counsellor herself was going through a prolonged and distressing episode, and knew that she needed to attend to aspects of her personal and domestic life which were undermining her work. It was the

consulting group that helped her decide to take action – more was not needed. The attentive, trusting atmosphere of the group made it easy, in fact quite natural, for her to report back about what she decided; *but* there would have been no need to do so, and probably (depending on how well everyone had got to know each other) *nor would they have asked* in subsequent sessions, because it was not then their business, unless the consultee had brought it back to the group.

The areas clarified were about her own self-management: from within, in her family, and about the possibility of regular supervision sessions. The group's assumption, this being consultation, not supervision or therapy, was that the counsellor was a competent professional and a competent person who needed only 'refloating' out of an overwhelming situation; it provided the right combination of (a) an accepting, calm setting and (b) the necessary questions to help her back on course again.

2 In the second case the problems, similarly resolved, were in the areas of the institutional history of the college where she worked, a number of its accepted practices which didn't now match what her job required, and the fossilisation of the old job, not only in her contract but in assumptions about her role. Once exposed to the light of day, the counsellor and her manager were able to make sure she had the tools her job required.

3 *But supposing the manager had not?* He might have been uninterested, uncomprehending, or said her requests were unnecessary or impossible to meet.

The appropriate next steps for the consultation would have been to help the consultee/counsellor to think through what she could do about that. Explain again in another way? Ask that someone else in the administration look at the matter? Find out what formal meetings would consider such issues for its agenda? If necessary, what outside advocacy could she enlist?

Just as the group would not have turned its hand to psychotherapy or marital guidance, nor should it try to push managerial, legal or political remedies; all this was for the consultee to 'take elsewhere', using her own competence and energy, not that of the group. Thus the group could carry on with other business, clarifying, questioning, prompting, suggesting and then rolling on, and maintaining a work-focused, businesslike atmosphere which did not inhibit bringing up matters that got in the way of the consultees' work, or making too much of a big deal about them.

It is quite characteristic that problems presented to the group as difficulties with a client, or attributed by the consultee to his or her own failings in counselling skills, turn out to be due to quite different matters, sometimes in their personal lives, sometimes in the way their work is organised, or how it is organised for them (Steinberg and Hughes 1987). The work described above was successful because the participants knew enough about family and personal dynamics, therapist–client relationships, work practicalities and administration to select out which mattered, and to touch upon each in sufficient depth, but with a light touch.

4   Readers unfamiliar with consulting with organisations might assume that the above problems should surely have been obvious from the start. Only, I would suggest, in the textbooks, or in training courses. In ordinary day-to-day work, all of us can be drawn into team and organisational denial and avoidance of facing solvable and relatively clear-cut problems which have become clouded and amplified by the feelings surrounding them. Of these, the most insidious is the belief that a properly professional and competent person should somehow be able to manage such things 'like everyone else does' with a mixture of instinct and magic and tolerance and not making a fuss.

5   Earlier I suggested how the idea of the anatomy and physiology of the human body, as if in the back of the clinician's mind, enables extremely fast scanning of all the possibilities. I do mean fast; a general practitioner – any good doctor – dealing with disabling or distressing but relatively minor matters all day, and then picking up a major disorder, is probably fast-forwarding through the tracks of thousands of mental algorithms faster than it takes to write this sentence down. My case for finding time for systems consultation is based on the same semi-automatic approach, but with psychodynamic, group dynamic and social and administrative systems being added to the fields being tracked.

6   Before leaving these examples of consultative sessions identifying items for other agendas, here is a far simpler example, taken from an inpatient unit's staff group run on consultative lines (Steinberg 1986b). The group had many 'relaxed' features, in style and because to accommodate the realities of the coming and going of staff in training and nursing rotas the participants differed considerably each week. However, there were fixed features to give it focus and establish trust: for example, it had a leader who was from outside the team (Foskett 1986), it started and ended on time, and its rules included there being no agenda, no minutes, no discussing of the group outside the group, and anything at all requiring decisions was to be taken off to the meetings where decisions were made: to the unit's ward round and clinical conferences, and to the unit's monthly management meeting. The group was thus free of all responsibilities except the vital one of reflecting thoughtfully, in detail and in depth, about a whole range of the unit's business – its staffing, its policies, the way it was run, relationships within the team and with the rest of the hospital and of course its relationships with patients and their families.

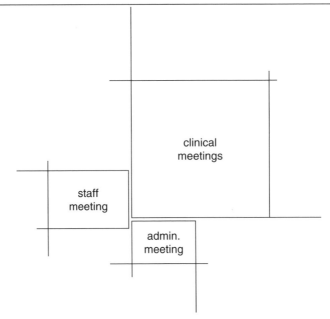

Figure 10: Three kinds of staff meeting.

The system of recognising three kinds of meetings: one clinical, one administrative and one immersed in the 'other' side of healthcare did seem to work to the advantage of all three meetings. And it worked both ways: chaotic matters coming up in ward rounds and the administrative meeting (e.g. conflict between staff) could be referred back to the staff meeting.

7 As I have identified *time* as a major resource and its proper use a neglected area, what about the time taken by all these meetings? The ward rounds and case meetings happened anyway as a necessity in the multidisciplinary team needed for a 28-bedded unit with extensive outpatient commitments. For the same reason, a unit management meeting was needed for internal policies and those relating to the rest of the hospital, and this busy meeting would last for around two hours every four to six weeks. The staff meeting happened weekly, for a strict 45 minutes. The time allotted for both non-clinical meetings therefore averaged under an hour and a half per week and seemed time well spent. But further research, as they say, is needed.

Example 7: consultation, not counselling (or psychotherapy)

We have already touched on this in previous examples. A general practitioner with psychodynamic psychotherapy training notices that an ordinarily conscientious and cheerful junior colleague is becoming uncharacteristically disorganised, stressed and bad-tempered. She suggests they discuss this after surgery one evening, and the two get into a prolonged conversation in which the younger doctor's obsessionality becomes evident as the key problem. She is having to double-check so many things so often that her work is becoming impossible to manage. The senior doctor suggests talking things over again, and on the second occasion a whole complex of matters begin to emerge: that the obsessional symptoms are an increasing problem outside work too and have only recently started to invade her professional life, that domestic life (which includes a busy husband and two small children) is now threatening to become destabilised too, and anxiety, depression, sleep disturbance and obsessive-compulsive symptoms are now chasing each other in a vicious cycle. But the doctor feels much better after their two conversations, her work begins to get back on an even keel, she says she will be fine, and that occasional conversations like these ones would be all she needs. The senior doctor has his misgivings about ad hoc meetings, and wonders about regular chats: not psychotherapy, but simply on a mentoring and monitoring basis.

The dramatic improvement is followed by a sudden deterioration again, and this time the junior doctor suggests the solution. She points out the complexity and wide ramifications of the problem – into her domestic life as well as her work, and back into her earlier history too. Plus other things she doesn't want to discuss with her colleague. The first two conversations helped her get things into perspective and now she feels she would like to see her own GP to discuss what kind of help is needed. However, they decide to use their good working relationship to meet briefly every so often to monitor how her symptoms are affecting her work, which will also help her decide what problems to prioritise with the outside cognitive behaviour therapist she is now seeing.

Comments

1   The woman doctor was right to suggest an alternative to her senior colleague's well-meaning efforts, suspecting correctly that his undoubted clinical skills would become unhelpfully blurred with all sorts of other sources of what Caplan (1970) identified as 'interference'. There was the friendly and informal working relationship which was welcome and useful in work, but would not be compatible with psychotherapy; in any case, she thought that systematic cognitive behaviour therapy and if necessary medication was indicated, and something along these lines was what she felt she preferred.

2   But she valued talking over with her senior from time to time the private but not too personal issue of how her symptoms affected her work, it not being that easy for a scrupulously careful professional in a

risk-laden field to know where to draw the line between being conscientious and over-conscientious. For the senior partner, he felt he could help monitor how his colleague was coping with stressful work, with permission and without being intrusive. The line between discussing her work and the complexities in the rest of her life was now clearly understood on both sides. These other parts of the system were relevant to her problem, but not to that aspect of it which was appropriate for their working relationship. Understanding about such complex systems was a necessary precondition to limiting what aspect they chose to deal with.

3   This was a potentially difficult situation finally well-handled on both sides. Note that the junior doctor, initially the consultee in her approach to her senior, took the lead in taking things in a different direction. This illustrates (a) the essentially peer–peer relationship necessary as a condition of consultation (notwithstanding their different status as doctors), (b) that being skilled and taking responsibility are part of the consultee's role too and (c) that where one starts out as consultant and the other as consultee, role-reversal should be no problem. These three important characteristics of the consultative approach highlight its fundamental difference from both hierarchical supervision and from psychotherapy.

4   Finally, in this example neither doctor need have particularly thought of themselves as formally undertaking systems consultation. It would have done no harm if they did; but it would be as good, to make again a point emphasised in this book, if the consultative approach could become second nature as another kind of professional conversation, and not only a particular set of techniques.

Example 8: consultation, not management

During staff group consultative sessions in a children's home, one of the newest members of staff, a forthright student on temporary training placement there, accuses a well-respected 'old hand' on the staff of regularly smelling of drink when he comes on duty. There are heated exchanges in the ensuing dispute, with some staff members embarrassed and silent and others taking sides, and among the accusations flying in both directions the student then says she also feels quite uncomfortable about the too intimate way the staff member relates to some of the youngsters at bedtime, eliciting an angry demand from the long-standing member of staff to explain exactly what she means. The visiting consultant knows they have got into a very important area: there is a real and potentially serious question to be handled here, but whether it is a matter of professional misconduct on the part of the regular staff member, or an inaccurate and inappropriate outburst on the part of a transient member of staff, or perhaps both, she can't say. At one extreme, disciplinary action or even police intervention might be needed; at the other, there could be an actionable accusation here.

Either way the staff group boat has been severely rocked, and the people present have to carry on working together meanwhile to contain a large group of severely disturbed children. The matter can't be dropped; but the rules guiding consultative work are being severely shaken here, because it isn't at this moment clear whether either the 'accused', or his 'accuser', is now meeting the criteria for peer–peer discussion, with properly and equally shared responsibility for handling whatever comes next.

The consultant says so. She calls a halt to the conversation, pointing out the seriousness of what's being said, and how it needs a different forum to resolve it. Certainly backtracking and apologies wouldn't resolve this matter. She says the meeting should continue to its allotted end, dealing as best they can with the unsafe and very troubled feelings that now exist all round, and in this respect they look at 'damage limitation' in terms of the rest of the day's and night's work. They discuss, as matters of fact, the machinery that exists within the children's home and its governing authority to deal properly with accusations of this sort and how to initiate it; and go on to see if guidance is needed for all present to respect the privacy of those involved without gossiping on the one hand or operating by denial on the other.

Comments

1   What suddenly erupted in the meeting wasn't consultative, but it needed to be dealt with, and thus the ground rules for consultation needed setting aside; it was right for the consultant to act with an authority ordinarily associated with a managerial meeting or some kinds of psychotherapy rather than consultation, using her own authority, responsibility and common sense as a professional worker. She also took some quick decisions that were to do with her understanding of the group dynamics of the place and the routine pressures and stresses within it.

2   Had the children's home Head been present, the consultant could have talked 'one-to-one' across the group to maintain his authority within the hierarchy of the Home, and – if necessary – consulted with him about both using the proper machinery for responding to the accusation and what to do about staff morale meanwhile. In his absence she encouraged discussion about what had happened in the group, acknowledging the crisis and the conflict between the different kinds of authority (*see* page 51) – hierarchical seniority, traditional authority and personal authority – as shown by different members of the group.

3   The consultant's work in this example also illustrates the potential for overlap at the boundaries of consultative work, therapeutic work and administration, as shown in Figure 3 (*see* page 14 *et seq*). The consultant conducted her work effectively through a sensitive understanding

of staff and group dynamics – but without conducting therapy – and of the requirements of administration – but without acting like a manager.

Example 9: training focus or work focus

A consultant in the care of the elderly with a clinical role at a care home is asked to take a consultative session about a very troubling medical and ethical problem concerning a resident. The staff learned a lot from the experience, particularly as it was focused on a current issue rather than a textbook topic, and asked if they could have further similar sessions. A series is arranged, with no 'curriculum' planned, but on each fortnightly occasion two of the staff members are invited to briefly present a problem or any other work issue that has arisen. These are used as the focus for the consultative session.

Comments

1 As illustrated in Figure 11 (*see* page 99), one of the strengths of this kind of consultative work is its dual capacity for teaching as it deals with a work issue, and dealing with a work issue by teaching. It thus represents one of the non-didactic approaches to teaching, and one where the consultant learns from the consultees about the world of work from their perspective. The first consultation was about a work crisis, the staff learning more from the experience than if they had simply been told what to do, or what they should have done. The subsequent consultative sessions were a contribution to in-service training, using day-to-day problems as the focus each time.

2 *But not only problems.* There is a 'third way' beyond (a) trusting that everything goes smoothly and (b) reacting to crises: that is, to anticipate the wider needs of the job. Thus, while another crisis would be a perfectly legitimate matter for the staff to bring up in their new and experimental training group, they could also raise, if they wish, anticipating questions such as how to handle relatives most helpfully, or how to get a better feeling for what it is like for an elderly and confused person to arrive in a new place. With growing experience and professional skills, consultees tend to move from crisis management to anticipating the finer points of their work (e.g. *see* Steinberg and Hughes 1987; Steinberg 1989a, 2000a), and to work proactively and preventively, rather than being primarily reactive.

3 On the same basis a team or organisation can ask for systems consultation to help guide them through a transition, whether chosen (e.g. a new kind of clientele or management style) or imposed (e.g. a closure, change or other development).

Example 10: the contract, and confidentiality

In Example 8 the children's home consultant had initially been asked to consult to the children's home over the telephone and in the vaguest of terms. Her name had 'come up', as she was told, because some months before she had handled an emergency there so helpfully, rather as with the experience of the geriatric physician in Example 9. The consultant suggested meeting the caller instead, who explained he was merely a go-between, and it would be better to meet X. However, despite the caller's promised arrangements, X never phoned. After a time, taking the matter seriously and at face value, she left a message at his office. Some weeks later Y called to say X had left, and what was it all about?

In the event Y suggested a meeting to discuss what had been wanted. At the meeting several people in different positions in the organisation requested outside consultation, although the consultant noticed that terms like 'staff support', 'supervision' and 'therapy' seemed to be used interchangeably. She described her own interpretation of consultation, and asked for a meeting with the Head of the children's home and its outside administrative supervisor, to see what they wanted and to explain what she could offer. She also took the opportunity to ask for confirmation of such matters as being paid and having travelling expenses reimbursed, which caused a characteristic flurry. Thus a contract was arranged.

Comments

1   Perhaps surprisingly, it is quite often like this, and would-be consultants are advised to follow the guidance given in this book for clarifying who wants what of whom, when and how, and how they will be paid for the service by the potential employer.
2   Almost always such apparent reliance on extrasensory perception is due merely to endemic muddle and misunderstanding; in general one can trust conversations with the right people, once tracked down, and then confirm a few points in an exchange of letters, rather than asking for a detailed contract. But vigilance is important, and for some longer term relationships with an organisation a proper contract is advisable.
3   For longer term agreements, e.g. more than a dozen meetings, I think it is wise to build in a review meeting as a definite point at which the progress and value of the sessions are considered. It can be useful to make no assumptions about continuing; one may consult the consultees about what has been helpful and unhelpful about the sessions, and similarly the pros and cons of continuing.
4   The organisation's management quite often perceive consultation, albeit that it is about learning how to do the job well, as something of a luxury extra. Staff on rotas may be 'drafted in' to make up numbers, or

asked to stay on at the end of the day, perhaps unpaid. The consultant should be aware of such things from the start, and be prepared for overstretched, undertrained, underpaid staff who genuinely appreciate the sessions and just as genuinely, and reasonably, prefer to get home on time and have their usual breaks. This development too can be anticipated, and if not dealt with right at the start, can provide a useful focus for a review session with the senior managers.

5   The practicalities of where, when and *how* to meet is important. There are residential settings where the need and motivation for such sessions is very high precisely because of the chaotic use of time and space that already prevails. Disturbed residents may cluster, hungry for attention, outside the room, where more staff than they have ever seen together are apparently relaxing in a circle of armchairs. And the phone will constantly ring. Will there be tea or coffee? Who will make it? And an early decision may have to be made about smoking.

6   Moving from the contract with the employers to the contract with the participants, matters like *attendance*, *gossiping* and *confidentiality* need to be raised. Regarding attendance, it is desirable but impracticable to expect all group members to attend every one of a series of groups. A useful principle borrowed from psychotherapy is that people speak only for themselves, and not about or on behalf of others or in broad general-isations. Such things can be discussed when they arise in the group, if not at the start of the first meeting. As they say, the usual conditions apply: consultation can only deal fully with matters for which those present can provide the necessary information, and for which they have some authority and responsibility; although as we shall see, some things can be partly dealt with, as in Example 1, where the limits of a parti-cular consultee's scope were pointed out, but she was helped to think through where to take the matter so that it could be properly consid-ered.

By 'gossiping' I mean that kind of wild chit-chat which is enjoyable for the participants partly because by its nature it relieves people of responsibility for accuracy or confidentiality, and which is a social activity, not a professional one.

In consultation, as in psychotherapy, language and communication are to be valued, respected and used seriously and with precision. When what sounds like gossip comes up in a consultative meeting the speaker should be invited to clarify the facts, which are either what he or she has observed, or what he or she has been made to feel.

For example, A may say that he finds B's style of organisation unclear or confusing, and this is acceptable because within the rules of consulta-tion, i.e. treating the consultee as a person of integrity, this (what he says he experiences) is presumed to be true. However, the bald judge-ment that 'B is a poor organiser' may not only be untrue, but by being one person's judgement offers the meeting nothing to discuss – except A's subjective judgement. Statements like 'I find B's conferences leave me feeling unsure what he wants me to do' may sound tortuous (and perilously like psychobabble), compared with 'B never gives clear instructions', but the former is a statement of fact from and about the speaker, and correspondingly something those present can work with.

Gossip includes discussing the content of a session outside the group. It can't be prevented, and is to an extent to be expected, but an ethos of discussing the group after it's over suggests a misunderstanding of what the group is for. One might as well casually continue a surgical operation outside the operating theatre, oblivious to the fact that the rest of the team have dispersed and the patient has woken up. That's how importantly a session devoted to systems consultation should be taken, and by the same token someone wanting to chat about the group after it is over should be asked to wait until the next meeting, unless it is claimed to be urgent, in which case it should be dealt with clinically or administratively, whichever is appropriate. All of which sounds rather po-faced and zealous, but we all natter all the time, and the serious task of consultative work needs to clear a definite time and space for itself.

As to confidentiality, people should feel free to bring what they wish to a consultative meeting – again, about facts – without it being repeated to others outside the meeting. One of the problems of a consultation group being mistaken for a 'therapy group' or 'support group' – which you will find regularly happens – is that the emotionally overburdened will think it is an opportunity to let it all hang out. It isn't. It is a self-disciplined, thoughtful and reflective piece of work. One way or another, things may be said about others which should not be said, and whether inappropriate, mistaken or not shouldn't be casually repeated elsewhere, unless of course they are matters to be formally and responsibly raised in the proper way, e.g. on a clinical or administrative occasion. Unless a group of staff have clearly developed a group ethos which respects confidentiality, the consultant should remind them of this at the outset.

Example 11: adapting the rules

A psychiatrist takes a staff consultation group at a large inner-city school which has many disturbed children from dysfunctional and deprived families. She adheres particularly carefully to the rules of working through the teaching staff's understanding and skills because of the importance of maximising staff confidence and independence. For example, when inattentive, overactive, misbehaving children are discussed she helps them explore their own ways of handling the children and working with parents, social workers, education social workers and the police. When some children remain problematic despite all these things being tried, she waits for the staff to ask if the child might benefit from something extra, for example behaviour therapy from a psychologist, or medication.

One day a particularly awkward and increasingly unpopular boy is presented as having violent and unpredictable outbursts despite all efforts, and the staff are divided over whether to keep trying with him or whether he should be suspended, although one or two staff confound this view by insisting he is a gentle, sensitive, if idiosyncratic child. One teacher says the boy is mad, 'ill', shouldn't be among ordinary kids, and ought to be seen in a clinic if not taken to hospital. The consultant often hears such comments, but this time thinks the teacher might be right. She asks a few clinical-type questions about the child, and as a result asks if the parents would like to arrange for him to be seen at her child psychiatric clinic, where she makes a diagnosis of schizoaffective disorder. He improves sufficiently on medication to return successfully to the school.

Comments

1 The consultant psychiatrist has changed gear from systems consultant to clinician because that is what the situation demanded, on clinical, ethical and not least on commonsense grounds. This represented bending one aspect of the consultative rules, but not entirely, because she could see that the common sense, descriptive, plain English of consultation wasn't sufficient in this child's case; she recognised the possibility of a true illness on clinical grounds, and was right to replace the 'consultative' with the 'clinical' in the circumstances.

2 This example of the inevitably fuzzy boundary between clinical and consultative work illustrates something useful about the consultative approach in a world where there is an ever-increasing clamour for diagnostic and treatment services. Consultative work proceeds as if the decision for a specialised, clinical approach is a socio-cultural decision rather than a purely clinical one, i.e. based on what front-line people (in this example, teachers and parents) cannot do, even with help, rather than because the symptoms and signs of illness are recognised. Clearly this route to clinical help is often not appropriate: appendicitis, meningitis, cardiac infarction and innumerable other conditions do need specialised recognition and specialised treatment, often swiftly. But health services do have an increasingly heavy commitment to a growing weight of vaguely defined and uncertainly determined conditions, sometimes 'psychosomatic', sometimes chronic, sometimes undiagnosable by traditional criteria, where it is far from clear whether what is needed is treatment, a change of lifestyle, a change of circumstances or even a different philosophy of life. The latter will include some things within the range of what 'ordinary' people outside healthcare should do

for each other and for themselves, and a case can be made for consultative work being what is needed to explore this possibility.

In this example, the clinician spotted illness, but in her particular consultative practice with the school, problems usually became psychological or psychiatric when the best commonsense efforts by teachers and parents couldn't achieve enough. This aspect of the philosophy of consultative work is discussed in Chapter 12, and also in Steinberg 1983 and 1989a and in Tyrer and Steinberg 2005.

3   In identifying a child as needing psychiatric assessment, the consultant was acting outside her contractual agreement. The right thing to do was to 'track back', as it were, so that one of the consultees (in this case the child's class teacher) could mention to the parents the consultant's question about their child and suggest they ask their GP for a child psychiatric referral. Depending on various circumstances, e.g. severity of illness and likely degree of anxiety, the psychiatrist could have had a word with the GP too, and perhaps offered to meet the child's parents with his teacher, to explain.

Concluding note

The 'proper channels' along which organisations and services run have a kind of linear logic. Dr A makes a diagnosis of B, and then makes a referral to Dr C at the hospital, where, after a period on the waiting list, Dr C and colleagues assess the diagnosis and prescribe treatment. The system often works. In this chapter, however, we have been interested in each step, rather than the stepping stones. Thus Dr A's feelings, thinking and reasoning, the nature and purpose of a 'waiting list', and what Dr C and colleagues anticipates and how they work together and with their clientele come into focus. It is as if we have taken the anatomy of the healthcare organisation's nervous system for granted – there it is, logically laid out and capable of being set out in a diagram – and instead examined its synapses, those highly complex and discriminatory nervous connections: us. We, healthcare workers, other professionals, and the patients, are the synapses in the organisation, and the focus of consultation is how these synapses process what comes before them: what they reject or ignore, what they hold up, what they divert, what they pass on, and what they understand, misunderstand and do in the process. Systems consultation provides a unique and I think interesting opportunity to recognise that the human synapses of organisations are capable of thought, feeling and discrimination, and capable of seeing in a wider perspective what they and the organisation are doing.

CHAPTER 7

Consultation as teaching and training

- Reciprocity between working and training.
  Examples:
- Team training and the lighter touch.
- Team training and the dynamic depths.
- Training in consultation – mapping it out.
- Team training with group painting.
- Team training and the art of making tea.
- Sculpting as revelation.

Introduction

Consultation teaches as it goes along. It assumes nothing except that the place to start from is that which the consultees already know. This may be the consultee's understanding and information about a matter, for example, in their place of work or in one of their clients. When the primary focus is teaching or training, you start with the consultee's knowledge, beliefs and attitudes. For example, in the consultative approach, if teaching behaviourists about Freud, pharmacologists about alternative therapy, theologians about Darwinism (and all these things vice versa) the consultative dialogue starts from the perspective and understanding of the trainee/consultee. The consultant learns too: about the consultees' information base and capabilities, about how they perceive and solve problems, how they feel and think, and always something new about the learning process.

Joint learning and teaching is essential in modern, complex societies where specialised and sometimes hyper-specialised people need to engage in collaborative work or at least shared understanding. This may apply at a highly technical level where, for example, it may be important for the designers and users of high-powered investigative or therapeutic techniques and equipment to collaborate with people who know what it is like to be subjected to it; while at a more informal level a teacher, however expert, should learn from students too; a trainee might have spent time working with traditional healers or shamans or in a deprived area or culturally idiosyncractic area (not necessarily abroad), or grown up in a country where elaborate health services were better ordered. The consultant/teacher can usefully be reminded, too, about what it is like to be a student. Consultees' own cultural backgrounds and, if appropriate and admissible (because the topic may cause more anxiety than sex and death), even the political views of trainees bring important perspectives to wider considerations of healthcare. Sometimes a mature student might have a training in psychology, engineering, literature, history, philosophy – or first aid. It is worth finding out. All this is to do with the trainee's attitudes, background and knowledge, but there are also different people's ways of understanding things, whether this too is cultural (for example Eastern and Western philosophical positions) or simply how different people learn. This too should be of interest to teachers. It is astonishing, to take one example, that the widespread unpopularity of mathematics and the difficulty of learning mathematical concepts is to a greater or lesser extent blamed on pupils and students instead of flawed teaching. It is also worth considering how much the polarity between, say, psychoanalysis and behaviour theory, or 'orthodox' *versus* 'holistic' medicine (at some cost to healthcare training and practise) is because different students and academics find their respective concepts unfamiliar, difficult or uncomfortable, rather than because of their relative merits.

Teaching how to use systems consultation while demonstrating systems consultation

As we have seen, one of the capabilities of systems consultation is its inherent circularity in that learning from problem solving is seen as one of its most important characteristics, whether the primary task is to solve a problem or to teach. If the primary task is to solve a work problem (or deal with a work issue), then whatever the outcome, consultant and consultees alike know better for next time. Conversely, if teaching or training is the main point of the exercise, taking a development or situation at work as the focus (a) keeps the session relevant and down to earth and (b) demonstrates that exploring how to handle a problem along consultative lines is a powerful way of learning. Further, (c) it usefully illustrates the Mandelbrot model of natural systems falling into repetitive patterns at successive levels (Mandelbrot 1977), so that even the smallest piece of activity can have wider implications and represent larger matters, as we shall see from the shenanigans involved in the exercise in Example 16 – 'Making the tea.'

As to the role systems consultation could occupy in schemes of training

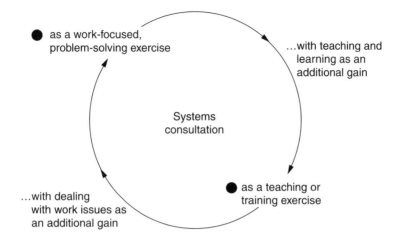

Figure 11: Circular relationship between systems consultation in training and as a work-focused exercise.

and learning in healthcare, I would place it alongside clinical skills or the 'bedside manner' (clinical – Greek *klinikos* – means 'bedside'). If the latter refers to the skills with which doctor and patient communicate, systems consultation starts out from how, for example, specialist, junior doctor, nurse, junior nurse, hospital chaplain, lab staff and other specialists communicate with each other across the bed; except that, in this book, we are looking at how to include the patient and relatives in this network too. Systemic consultation is therefore one of the three primary ways of conversing in healthcare, the other two being didactic and/or instructive, and clinical and/or therapeutic.

Example 12: an inter-departmental consultation: one way of beginning

A training seminar on improving communication between adult and child psychiatric services in psychiatry (a live issue in the hospital). I note the poised notebooks and the general air of expectation that the visiting lecturer will be imparting some wisdom. Instead of launching into a PowerPoint, bullet point presentation ('Communication = Concept, Contact, Clarity and Conciseness' or some such thing), I ask if anyone would like to tell me about a recent example of liaison between the two departments. As the teaching occasion I am thinking of took place in a relatively hierarchical, deferential culture, I dealt with the hush by kicking off with some experiences of my own, and then invited one or two of the senior people present if in turn they would like to describe a clinical case vignette illustrating the seminar's theme. What was described was very appropriate, some examples

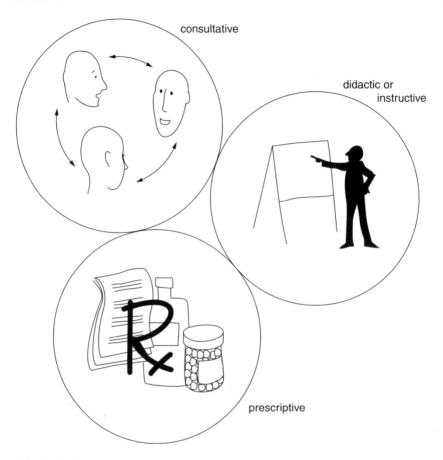

Figure 12:   Kinds of communication.

of the transfer of teenagers who had been admitted in an emergency over-night or at weekends to the very traditionally run adult wards, and then transferred in a day or two to the young people's service which relied more on psychotherapeutic and family work and less on drugs, and where multi-disciplinary work was more comprehensively established. However, frosti-ness, conflicts and disagreements between the two teams involved were only hinted at. There were also very occasional transfers in the other direc-tion, when an adolescent became very disturbed and was transferred for closer observation or containment or sometimes the monitoring of medica-tion like lithium or antipsychotic drugs, with which the adult nursing staff were more familiar.

By taking for granted and acknowledging the positive sides of the way the teams helped each other, it wasn't too difficult to suggest the kinds of problem that I thought might be there, because they are universal and prac-tically inevitable. Also, by deliberately taking a lead myself, while relating particularly (though not exclusively) to the seniors in the group, I hoped I had made it feel safe to touch on disputes, and that to discuss them in front of more junior staff and non-doctors, *and* in front of a guest (me) was acceptable.

What became alright to mention included, for example, confusion over who was in charge of the teenager's case during an untidy transfer, or 'difficulties' about a transfer in either direction. This was often identified in terms of bed availability, but (as I knew) also likely to involve mutual suspiciousness, competition and resentment between teams, or that peculiar strain between two hierarchies when the top and bottom people are in agreement but the middle grades find difficulties because they are closer to them. I simply described my own experiences in such things and one or two began to describe theirs. From this new position we could identify from the discussion important undercurrents, for example that a unit oriented to taking action in emergencies has a different set of procedures and lines of communication to one dealing with long-term feelings, relationships and family systems. Thus the transfer of care was *likely* to be problematic (indeed, it was surprising that it wasn't more so). We were then able to have a useful teaching session on the various levels of problem likely to be seen when patients had to be cross-referred. (This example is continued in Example 15.)

The session ended with a compromise between the tying up loose ends characteristic of didactic teaching, and the tendency in group dynamic work to deliberately leave things in the air. We spent the last quarter of an hour seeing how far the session had addressed the matters the participants had hoped it would; what had made the session consultative rather than didactic; and what would happen next, in the scheduled follow-up session after coffee, and – going briefly round the group – whether each had found anything, however minor, they might adopt in their future work. These aspects of closing a session *do* I think merit bullet points:

- feedback about the session
- comments on its particularly consultative perspective
- what if anything might be worth 'taking away'
- how to use the next session.

Systems consultation as a linguistic style

I hope it is clear from what has been said already that proposing consultation as a conversational style does not mean the adoption of mystifying jargon and other special language. Rather, it implies a readiness and ability to converse in plain language about the nuts and bolts of who is trying to do what with whom, why, and whether it is working. But having said this, there is a lot to be said for using non-verbal approaches as well, at least as a supplement, and this is the focus of the examples that follow, because speaking plainly about professional work and relationships and the feelings involved isn't necessarily easy, and if it seems easy it may not represent them accurately or fully enough.

The problem with group discussion alone is that it can revert to type and become a straight (linear) intellectual seminar, and the point of consultation is that it has a wider scope, tapping into more complex areas of people (personnel, clientele) and organisations. While psychotherapists sometimes try to identify the non-discussable by raising the emotional temperature and encouraging confusion as a starting point, consultation tends to use non-verbal strategies, some quite simple (e.g. diagrams), to find out about the 'wiring' of a system – who communicates with whom, where the lines of authority and control go, how many systems might be posing as one, and who might be left out of the system altogether.

There is another reason for trying to sidestep linear logic and formal discussion. Complex arrangements, whether in the way a department, a hospital or a country is run, are usually wreathed in mystery and mystification. This need not be a conspiracy on the part of those on the peaks, but simply the chaotic way organisations grow and consolidate themselves. No one person, not even the boss, quite knows what goes on, and this impenetrable structure characteristically provides a solid base that may allow minor changes and modifications but not major or radical ones. As with an individual's psychological denial, it is not a matter of dishonesty but a matter of maintenance by not probing, by not asking too many questions, by averting the gaze from uncomfortable, unproductive or unyielding areas. The same goes on in organisations, and it is cemented firmly together by the language and taboos of the place: some things aren't said, asked or even thought. Exploring this requires a different kind of tool on the consultative probe, and it is primarily non-verbal.

Ways of getting at the non-obvious

I have referred to strategies used in consultative work to raise the temperature and in a sense raise the stakes as a way of eliciting, as if by pathways alternative to the usual ones, some of the emotional issues that enable teams and organisations to get stuck in attitudes and procedures that seem undesirable, in rational terms, but mysteriously fixed – rather like neuroses. That style of consultation which leans towards the psychotherapeutic operates as if raising group tension and the group temperature melts some of the glue that causes inflexibility, thereby enabling new learning and change. One of the more powerful arguments for it is that it is more effective in bypassing routine, over-rationalised ways of thinking and talking about matters which have important emotional undercurrents. It has its place, particularly in training for consultative work, and for trainees or consultees already familiar with this kind of strategy or wanting to learn it; however, its predominantly affective approach is a limiting factor for a set of strategies which should be widely understandable, accessible and acceptable, and which start from where a wider range of potential consultees have got to so far in their work and training experience. Moreover, as discussed later, I would like to see a further step in which consultative techniques could be used readily in work with our patients and clients too. This kind of universal application would require consultative approaches to be readily comprehensible and user-friendly to whoever wants to use them. I also have the idea that work and learning about work could be fun.

Example 13, however, is an account of a consultative session leaning towards the more psychotherapeutic school of consultative work. The other examples in this chapter are ways of working which I believe are more accessible and more clearly focused on what the consultees bring for consultation, and closer to their own terms rather than to the conceptual models of the consultants. However, it is a subject open to argument, and my own preferred approach which is perhaps more like *play* is of course a conceptual model too.

Example 13: a training consultation in psychodynamic mode

A training session billed as an introduction to consultation begins in complete silence. There have been mutual introductions at an earlier session. People file in for a few minutes more and take their seats. There are curious and expectant glances in the direction of the training consultant, who gazes impassively at the opposite wall. Minutes pass, periods of silence alternating with shuffling. As this is abroad, there is also a little whispering. More people come in. After about 10 minutes there is a high level of perceptible tension, and some members of the group seem quite uncomfortable. One bold man asks if the session has started, and the teacher asks the group if anyone would like to answer him, though no one does.

There is a co-consultant, who was billed as introducing the subject, and he has been looking around the group with bright but non-committal interest, and then looking out of the window. He is now looking at a sheet of paper on his lap. After a time, someone asks 'are we going to start?' and the co-consultant looks up, surprised, and gives a kind of half shrug. Then the first consultant addresses the group, says how upset she is, because four or five people drifted in late. This has made beginning the group very difficult for her. The other consultant takes the cue, and says he had been expected to say a few words, but didn't now know what to say. This organisation – the group – was in difficulties, he points out. The latecomers have surprised and confused him. He had thought they would be interested. One of the latecomers, sitting awkwardly with his coat on his lap, attempts a reassurance that they are interested but the serving of lunch had been delayed. He apologises. The two consultants continue gazing at a point somewhere above the middle of the group. The meeting proceeds in fits and starts from there, and something is learned about what it feels like to be in a Kafkaesque setting whose purpose and procedures and mutual feelings are unclear and disrupted. Unfocused anger, disappointment and anxiety is expressed, and a number of participants who have clearly worked in group therapy make comments like 'I wonder why the group is so uncomfortable?', although the remarks are not taken up. Near the end, each consultant makes comments of their own, about structure and feelings of unsafety; people begin to join in, but the clock hands reach the hour just as one speaker is pausing between observations, at which point the consultants leave.

Comment

I can see what this kind of session is getting at in group analytical terms, and it has its place in psychodynamically-oriented group training, but I don't recommend it for general consultative work and training. However, it has its adherents, and a kind of rationale in emotionally-led learning, the guiding principle being living it rather than thinking about it. I find that some proponents of this way of working are not clear about the difference between consultation and therapy, and some maintain that there is no difference that matters. It is a strategy that as a student in the field you may come across from time to time, and it may or may not be what you want. Consult the consultant to find out how he or she approaches his work; be prepared for a response along the lines: 'I wonder why you ask?'

Example 14: consultation with diagrams: the value of charting a course

A training seminar in systems consultation for psychiatric specialist registrars begins with one of the SpRs presenting something from the past week's work. It has three aims: primarily, to teach an aspect of systems consultation by using an example of work; second, to help the SpR with that aspect of work; third, to look at the group teaching process itself – the practicalities as well as the dynamics. Teaching consultation, helping with a work issue, and teaching about teaching, are combined in one session, the balance between them varying from meeting to meeting.

The SpR presents an aspect of his liaison work with a large specialist clinic dealing with a chronic and relapsing physical disorder in children. He has only recently started there, but thought that by now he would have established a useful working relationship between psychiatry and the specialty, which he hasn't, and there is a history of no previous SpR ever feeling they achieved this; and yet it was the specialist department which asked for this kind of psychiatric input, and consistently makes it clear how very much it values it and wants it to continue. Thus we have an interesting mystery to solve.

First step: clarifying roles, lines of authority and communication

The SpR is asked by the group to describe the clinic, and a typical example of his liaison work, and this takes us straight in at the deep end. The clinic is a muddle, and there is no typical piece of work. The way the clinic operates means that the opposite number with whom he takes the joint clinic, a general physician, is different each week, and may be a consultant, SpR, research worker or visiting specialist trainee, is often a part-timer, and is sometimes a locum. Each expects something different from the SpR, and quite often nothing at all. Sometimes he feels treated like a senior specialist, sometimes like a student. The patients, even those attending frequently, vary in a similarly kaleidoscopic way, thus each patient presents his or her child's chronic problems afresh, and the SpR has observed and tried to comment on some quite substantial resultant changes in the advice and approach taken. However, the patients and families, some of whom travel quite a long way, and most of whom have a very long wait to be seen, seem very happy with the service. Two of its features are a circulating tea trolley manned by a couple of exceptionally chatty and cheerful volunteers, and the senior physician, Dr A, who seems to amble at will from his own clinic in and out of the sister's and senior social worker's offices and around the other doctor's desks. He seems to know all the patients, and they him. Another feature of the clinic is a stream of clinical visitors who the SpR has seen there before and who drop in to see the doctors there, occasionally borrowing a desk to deal with – presumably – last week's notes and letters. There is for the most part a warm and friendly buzz, except for the secretaries and filing staff who hasten around in, so it seems, a state of tight-lipped frenzy. The SpR says it feels like a cross between a club and an old-fashioned marketplace.

The SpR doesn't know how it all works, whether it is 'all right' or eccentric, and doesn't know how he fits in or what he should do – except that the clinic seems happy with his input. He has been trying to find out about it for himself, mostly by chatting to the succession of doctors and the senior social worker, and as he describes it he draws a plan or map of sorts of the clinic, including a kind of family tree of who's who. The 'map', redrawn and revised in the light of the group's questioning, is quite revealing, Figures 13 and 14 giving 'before' and 'after' impressions of the scene as it gradually becomes clarified.

There are two sources of authority. One is the Academic Unit, which supplies large numbers of middle grade and visiting academics, many part-time and briefly visiting from overseas, and it seems often quite well established in their fields with many publications to their names. It provides, the group concludes, rather impressive technical authority. The other is Dr A, the very senior clinician, well known in the hospital and worldwide, who provides traditional authority, though this seems shared with the senior social worker, and one of the senior nursing sisters, who is also supposedly his girlfriend. It seems that she looks after him and his own staff, and the other nursing sister, a clinical nurse specialist, looks after the academic staff. It seems that no communication between these two hierarchies is looked for in the running of the clinic.

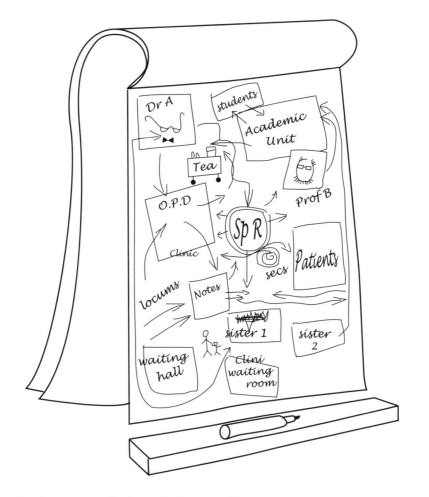

Figure 13: En route to clarification and looking impossible.

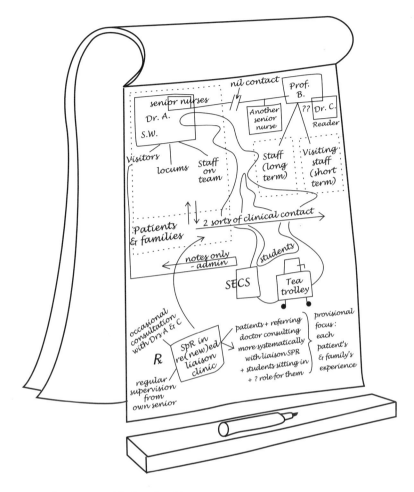

Figure 14: Still en route and looking feasible.

The layout of the clinic, straddling the edge of the main outpatient building, a small courtyard backing onto the kitchens and some linked Portakabins, reflects the main groups. The history of the clinic included the academic unit needing a large and busy clinic for its middle grade research staff to have available for clinical experience and research (their output is first class), something the senior physician, probably nearing retirement (but likely, it is thought, to then be his own locum) is happy to help with. There are grumblings about the clinic, it seems, from the administration, whose secretaries have to deal with considerable chaos, and from medical students and student nurses, who get little systematic teaching, but the senior clinical and academic staff seem happy with the way things run, and so it seems are the patients, indeed a respected self-help organisation has a thriving branch here. The senior physician is its patron.

The role of the liaison SpR is not clear. It was requested by the clinic's seniors about three years before, following a peak of dissatisfaction from elsewhere in the hospital about what was perceived as a highly idiosyncratic and old-fashioned arrangement. A consultant psychiatrist nearing retirement acted as liaison psychiatrist for a time, and the job then became one for her rotating SpRs. Supervision of the SpR's work by the retired consultant psychiatrist's successor has not yet been set up.

The clinic seemed to have achieved a kind of homeostasis between old-fashioned medicine and cutting-edge research, with no complaint, still less any evidence of dissatisfaction, from its clientele. The most junior of the students seemed to gain nothing very much, and the secretaries and their assistants seemed to pay the highest price in various ways for their role in the engine room of this odd vessel. The SpR fantasised that indeed if anything were done to threaten its modus operandi, its patients might well rise up in mutiny.

Step 2: clarifying the liaison SpR's role

First, the group clarifies for the SpR how the role confusion in the clinic has been undermining his clarity about his own role; dodgy boundaries don't affect one side only. He is, moreover, a particularly conscientious sort of person who prefers his work to be well-ordered. A sub-theme is that the SpR was wondering whether he had some kind of ethical or professional responsibility to act in some way on the deficiencies he perceives in the way the clinic is run. The group decides not, or at least not directly, because it seems that there is already controversy in the hospital administration about this.

However, he would be expected to make some kind of representation if he couldn't do his own liaison job properly; and the group's attention is now focused on (a) what he is expected to be doing, (b) whether he can and (c) what supervision he gets in this work. The group discusses the third point first and the SpR agrees that he should ask his own consultant to provide regular opportunities to discuss his liaison work.

The existing arrangement for liaison work is that the two or three middle grade doctors seeing the patients refer people with possible problems to the 'liaison clinic', which means the SpR and whichever other doctor he is working with each week. However, the ad hoc doctor–patient contact the clinic favours doesn't enable the SpR to do his job with any continuity, and it is concluded that he should suggest a more suitable arrangement. He will in future *write* to the referring doctor a note about his conclusions *and* ask to see the same patient again with that doctor after an appropriate interval. First, however, he will discuss this proposal with his own consultant and then write to the two people who, according to the 'discoveries' of the flip charts, are in clinical charge – the senior consultant, Dr A, and, as it turns out when enquiries are made with Professor B, the Reader in Medicine, Dr C. The letter invites a meeting to discuss this, if wished, and a review meeting after three months to see how the new arrangement has been working and who has been seen. In the group two weeks later, the SpR is able to report that the Reader in Medicine thought the idea excellent and agreed with the plan, if the senior consultant did too, which was the case. In fact Dr A said he had been wondering how the 'psychiatric side' had been going. However, while he agreed with the principle of introducing some predictability into the follow-up for psychiatric purposes, he had misgivings about whether the secretaries and the appointments and filing staff could handle the new style of working. This, it was decided, would be for Dr A to sort out in some way with his team.

Comments

1 A chart or diagram of who is involved in an organisation and their respective positions, literally and metaphorically, can be useful in clarifying complex arrangements. (Sculpting, described in Example 17, takes this a step further.)

2 The consultation session used the chart and other means simply as an attempt to describe what was happening, which is a basic first step in systems consultation. What to do about any of it was another matter, but not one which could be addressed amid the confusion. Allowing confused situations to develop or continue is commonly found as a strategy to inhibit examination and change.

3 The confusion was treated here as the responsibility of the people who, despite it all, seemed to be in charge. The SpR's decision to make at least his contribution clear and systematic was primarily so that he could get on with his part of the job. However, changing this very small part of the system (if allowed to happen) can sometimes act as the kind of adjustment within the machinery that changes other parts of the system too. For example, it would not be possible to meet the SpR's request unless the secretaries and filing staff are allowed to change their ways of working, and this in turn will not happen unless the people overtly or otherwise managing the clinic declare their responsibilities and authority and find some way of negotiating with the administrative staff. At the same time three senior people (Dr A, Dr C and the SpR's own senior) had been reminded of their roles.

4 This step fulfilled one of the rules of systems consultation: the SpR acted *as if* the nominal seniors would act with authority and responsibility. If they can't or won't, this brings up a new set of questions; for example, can they use liaison psychiatry?

5 The training group, practising and teaching consultation as it went, had to negotiate a course that took account of whether particular ways of

working were good or bad, ethical or unethical, or professional or unprofessional, without making these issues the primary focus. The purpose of the group was to help the SpR in his work and to teach, not to hold an inquiry into other people's working practices. Correspondingly, it allowed for personal feelings and personalities (e.g. the SpR's orderliness, which might have surprised some of the clinic staff) without questioning them or suggesting they be modified. Again, the autonomy of the SpR was taken for granted here too.

6 But supposing the SpR had held ethical views at great variance with the work of the clinic, making his work impossible. (Suppose for example it dealt with termination of pregnancy, to which the SpR objected.) Then the systems consultation frame (or goalposts) would have to shift again, and the new question raised would be not whether the clinic should change but whether the SpR could work there; and again, suppose his position was that *no one* should work in a clinic like that; then that is yet another issue, and the purpose of consultation should then shift to helping him decide what to do about it. Thus the focus shifts as necessary to stay with a consultative role, not a quasi-managerial or hierarchical one.

7 The SpR was encouraged by the group to ask for supervision of his liaison work by his consultant to be set up. The absence of adequate supervision is a common finding in many fields when systems consultation explores why someone is in difficulties in their work. This is one of the many examples in consultative work where examining the details of a single piece of work can demonstrate wider issues at another level, particulary the common assumption that once qualified and given a job description, most health and care workers can get by without work-focused supervision. For workers with more seniority, experience and responsibility (e.g. newly appointed consultants or their equivalent in other fields), mentoring has been recommended in recent years, and the consultative approach would seem to be a good model for it.

8 Was the clinic 'good' or 'bad'? The SpR and the group were rather exercised by this. Remember Klein and Robin Skynner (*see* page 45); in reality, many things are a mixture of the good, the bad and the mediocre, the pressure to categorise into black and white coming from the kind of brain and mind we have. Questions concerning ethics and values are appropriate for a consultative training group, but should follow consultation's analysis of the details of the whole of what actually happens, rather than making superficial assumptions. The view of the Reader in Medicine was that the clinic operated along some rather chaotic and outdated lines, but the senior physician seemed to know all the patients and what was going on with all of them; and they in turn seemed to like the clinic and his benignly autocratic style. These are deep waters.

Example 15: a group painting as an exercise in systems consultation

This example represents a further stage in the consultation session described in Example 12. There, conflict between two psychiatric units which needed to collaborate was interpreted not as a clash of personalities but as the result of quite different ways of working. For example, the adult psychiatric ward tended to work on traditional medical lines, with linear concepts of causality (e.g. metabolic upset causing depression, in turn causing suicidal behaviour) and treatment in wards with medication, while the young people's unit used family and other social concepts in its understanding of the teenagers, and family therapy, educational methods and psychotherapy as well as drugs. Also, the very stretched adult unit had to work on a quick admission, quick discharge principle, while the unit for adolescents needed as far as possible to plan its admissions carefully with the family and the ward, and similarly to prepare its young people for discharge home. Each service needed the other: the adult psychiatric service didn't feel prepared for working with young people, nor were its wards suitable; while the young people's unit couldn't maintain a therapeutic environment for children while taking in unprepared emergencies round the clock. But this rational side to the debate did not prevent the adult services perceiving the adolescent service as fussy, selective, a bit delicate and not really pulling its weight, especially over emergency admissions; while the adolescent service perceived the adult service as too narrowly medically oriented, too tough-minded and restrictive, and with neither its diagnoses nor its treatments matching the children's needs. There were many occasions when the busy adult ward had to plead with the adolescent service to hurry up and take a patient; and, when the adolescent ward was full, there were times when the adolescent service wanted a young patient admitted as an emergency but could not provide one of its own beds. It was a real (and very common, worldwide) clash of therapeutic cultures, compounded by a blurring of who was in charge of each child's case during emergency periods, and confused by different attitudes among the staff; for example a few adolescent unit workers thought the brisk adult approach was just what the teenagers needed, and some adult unit workers admired and envied the slower, more reflective and more broadly therapeutic style of the other team.

But stating all this would be merely to state what everyone already knew, and in any case 'rational' discussions had ended in deadlock because the differences were ones of background, attitude and temperament and not really mutually comprehensible. So instead, in the second session, when key staff from both teams were somewhat more relaxed and felt that a number of things which needed to be stated to each other had been said, I suggested that the two teams spend the rest of the day doing a joint painting on these themes.

This kind of task can cause apprehension for those unused to it, particularly for those who learned early in school that 'they couldn't draw'. It can leave people feeling as if performing, judged and exposed. In addition, an art session seems to be taking a turn towards 'play' rather than real adult work and talk, and this can cause apprehension and embarrassment.

As discussed in Chapter 11, this is actually part of the rationale of using art work alongside or instead of talk – participants are then using new ways of conceptualising ideas and communicating them, well away from the familiar kinds of thinking, talking and behaviour of the usual sort of meeting or conversation. This provides opportunities for innovation and new thinking; but it also feels potentially unsafe. Whoever takes a session along these lines has a professional obligation to establish trust and make the setting safe enough for new exploration (see for example the notes on attachment theory, and Winnicott's 'facilitating environment', page 47, and Steinberg 1991).

Acknowledging all this and taking responsibility for this approach (not the outcome) was part of the atmosphere I would want to develop early in exercises like this. There are various ways of getting people involved unselfconsciously in creative and 'action' techniques, and these are perhaps a distraction from the focus of this book. One simple step for establishing safe-feeling boundaries is to outline the day's timetable, including coffee breaks and how and when the day's work will end. It is also important to suggest a clear task, a way of beginning, and do so briefly. What participants then make of it is up to them. The task here was to use paintings or sketches in any way they liked to make a large-scale plan of the two units and their interconnections, using images and symbols rather than labels. The materials provided were lots of thick felt-tip pens, watercolours and brushes, and eight sheets of A3 paper sellotaped together to form a giant blank sheet spreading across several tables.

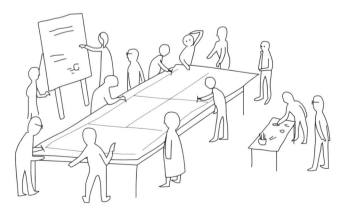

Figure 15:   Group painting. Subject: a plan of the relationship between two units.

On this occasion I left writing, drawing and painting as the main options for communication, rather than the only medium, and suggested the minimum of discussion of the sort we had had earlier. One task however, an attempt to provide a channel for the strictly verbal plus a kind of memorandum, was that key words or phrases that occurred to people as they got on with painting could be written on a blackboard at any time as an agenda for the discussion which was to end the day: words and phrases like 'families', 'pulled two ways', 'pressure', 'night staff', 'control', ' communication', etc.).

This exercise was productive and useful, and during it some participants initially on the sidelines joined in with more enthusiasm. The drawings included quite a lot of jokes and cartoon images, and simple decorations, with arrows indicating relationships. The adult department was represented by such images as people in white coats wielding syringes, a grand entrance with rows of steps, and rows of beds, a figure who turned out to be the boss taking a ward round, and a large car park at the front with ambulances cruising through the lanes. Telephone wires ran all over the place between various parts of the adult area and the adolescent unit, which was represented by both teams as bunches of brightly dressed young people lying about, sitting hunched up or fighting (or playing?) with the staff, and faces with broad grins or lots of turned down mouths. There were also flashes of lightning coming out of dark clouds on the adolescent unit's side, and ECT machines issuing sparks on the adult side. Various exercises included each team 'visiting' the other to see how their part of the painting was going, and then swapping paintings to add their own bits to the other's work. There was also a pause for questions and discussion about the images. Someone wanted to draw in the whole, parent hospital, and this became a joint exercise and took the form of a kind of castellated maze which embraced the adult psychiatric unit but left most of the young people's unit (a more recent development) out. Someone drew adolescent staff lying back and reading in bed, and at a picnic, while adult unit staff were pictured in old-fashioned uniforms. There was a (suggested) attempt to draw in pictures and images of things that would make mutual relationships better, and although this was not very successful on paper, it led into an animated debate.

The main conclusion was to plan a meeting with key staff from both units plus representatives from one or two other hospital departments, which appeared in the drawing as looking more involved with some of the emergent issues than had been expected; for example, from Administration and the School of Nursing. This meeting turned out to be better prepared and more productive than previous crisis-focused meetings had been, and a further one was planned.

Comments

1   It could be argued that the afternoon of using art had been more like play, with nothing like all the expected big issues discussed. It was certainly relaxed, with alternating periods of silent, intense work and amusement. The approach through art had highlighted some unexpected issues (like who worked where, and what it was like) and played down some very specific agenda items some had expected (e.g. 'what to do with a young person on the borderline between each unit's age ranges'). I think what had been achieved was not the solution to a hundred detailed 'issues' but a better working relationship between the two teams and a fuller picture not only of what work was like for the other department, but of the wider connections and ramifications of their own. Those of us interested in the broad sweep of what goes on in healthcare services can easily forget the narrow perspective forced on people who have to rush in and out of part-aspects of the work, e.g. night staff who often have little real opportunity even to hear about some of the activities of the day. As we have seen in other examples, crucial roles are sometimes thrust on under-trained, low status and part-time people, and the insights of staff in such positions, when they are given the chance to express them, can be eye-opening for senior people who thought they knew how the system operated.

    But whatever such revelations, the fact of the group event happening at all was a revelation in itself, showing that working relationships and practices and the experience of being a member of staff were worthy of reflection. For many people this was quite new.

2   Such events can feel unfamiliar and unsafe, particularly where hierarchical and disciplinary boundaries are suspended to an extent, and providing a definite timetable (with tea and coffee breaks) and a basic guide to the day's activities frees people to experiment and 'play' within them. Play is a serious matter, as everyone from evolutionary biologists to court jesters know. Visual jokes, cartoons and funny drawings produced quantities of material for discussion that could never have been placed on a formal agenda.

3   The main organisational outcome was a subsequent and much more productive 'serious' meeting between the departments, plus one or two other departments 'discovered' in the group painting to have important roles. However, it did seem that positive changes had in any case already occured among staff on both units: another area for research?

Example 16: party game: who will make the tea?

This provocative and informative exercise examines decision making, roles and authority in multidisciplinary teams. The explosive charge is placed by dividing a large group into into four or five subgroups which are likely to be of unequal size, for example doctors, nurses, psychologists, social workers and secretaries. It is then announced to universal consternation that there has been a problem in the catering department, and that they will have to provide coffee and tea for themselves in the next short break. Each group is asked to put aside the scheduled discussion of interdisciplinary decision-making for a few moments while, in their own group and (if they wish) in liaison with other groups they organise tea, coffee, milk, sugar, hot water, cups, spoons, trolley, porterage, washing up, etc.

Comments

1   Quite probably an open and non-hierarchical atmosphere will have developed for this training occasion, a trap into which the group may fall. The result can provide food for thought about hierarchical and cross-disciplinary working and decision-making.
2   The exercise is more like a party game than a role play, in that there is usually a bit of subversion by some to make sure an easy and unlikely option isn't chosen, e.g. by the doctors volunteering to make the tea. (This might be countered by the psychologists, say, asserting that they would. No competent organisation, after all, will want the same job duplicated.) The task is to negotiate: but with a little sabotage (which may seem like mischief, but in fact is quite close to some of the subterranean activities which happen in teams) group participants tend not to fall into the customary patterns of compromise and letting things pass that normally prevail. And how is it decided whose approach will be adopted?

Example 17: sculpting roles: who's close to whom?

Sculpting is a dramatherapy technique and should be conducted by people experienced in using it and familiar with the principles and practice of dramatherapy and role play in general (Jennings 1987). Brudenelle's account (1987) of work with people with learning impairment is I think a good introduction, partly because of her approach to the subject, but also because people taking part for the first time in activities like dramatherapy or role play can find it a new and unsettling experience. It is indeed like having to learn a whole set of unfamiliar ways of being and behaving, and can be useful for illuminating aspects of what goes on in a working group or team (Brudenelle 1987; Jennings1987).

The exercise begins with simple steps designed to encourage mutual trust, and may well have followed a number of other activities (like making the tea!). The person taking the group may invite one of the participants to be a co-worker and to act as a focus for the sculpt – for example as a client of a clinical team, or its secretary.

The essence of a sculpt is that people take up positions that represent themselves in relation to others. The positions include body posture and the direction of gaze as well as where they place themselves in the room. They may or may not choose to look at particular people, or to touch them, and they might to a limited extent move, e.g. looking from A to B and back again, or for example holding X away from themselves while beckoning to someone else.

In one exercise involving a multidisciplinary team there was a most dramatic static scrum in which everyone wanted to hang onto and be close to two key clinical figures and the part-time secretary (who managed to convey her part-time status brilliantly by regularly coming and going from the room). Two people – a senior doctor and a senior nurse – who needed to be close to (in touch with) each other were physically prevented from doing so because of the tight circle of people surrounding each of them.

People were asked to maintain this sculpt for a reasonable and humane period while volunteering how it felt, and also whether this felt like their position in work. Feelings (later listed as an agenda for later, as in Example 15) included quite high levels of apprehension, frustration and tension, which felt 'OK' in the sculpt but were remarkably similar to similar feelings in the day's work which were decidedly not OK; these feelings were often related to such experiences (in the sculpt) as 'trying to keep an eye on C, D and E while being within reach of F, G and H but close to J and K at the same time'. Everyone wanted easy access to the secretaries, who again were hemmed in by some participants, while others who indicated their occa-

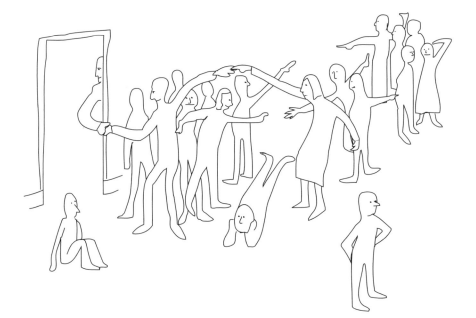

Figure 16: A revealing 'sculpt'.

sional need to be in touch with them couldn't get near them. Those who seemed to have the most peripheral and erratic contact with some team members were sometimes participants taking the role of its clientele.

The consultant taking the group didn't know the team well but was able, from the sculpt, to give some remarkably accurate guesses about what the working team was ordinarily like. Starting with the person acting as co-worker and focus, people were then asked to try to get into a physical position that 'felt better'. This proved easier for some than others. The consultant's co-worker also stood in for people – i.e. adopted their position – allowing them to step outside their place and posture and take a look at it in relation to the whole. People were also invited to try other people's positions, to see how they felt.

After a break people discussed what the experience had been like and how it related to their work. Where people have adopted another's role, time should be allowed for them to 'de-role'.

Comments

1   The technique can produce a remarkably accurate and useful picture of working relationships and the kind of feelings emerging from them.
2   The procedure can begin as rather enjoyable fun, and certainly a relief from trying to describe working relationships in words, but then lead to quite intense feelings of frustration, confusion and helplessness, and of the 'impossibility' of some tasks and roles, feelings which do require experienced handling.
3   As with other creative techniques, the experience is likely to reveal connections, disconnections and relationships which hadn't been particularly noticed before, and this can be useful for rethinking the actual ways people relate to each other at work, for example, when trainee and supervisor can't actually meet regularly because of work demands on both. However, as with Example 15, the outcome is not only about specifics, but an opening up of other ways of thinking about one's own work and implications for administration and training.

Consultation as supervision

Earlier I have stressed the importance of not confusing hierarchical supervision with consultation. Supervision within training can be consultative in style or essentially hierchical, both having their place. There is a role, little used in medical training though routine in psychotherapy and counselling, for regular, systematic case discussion on consultative lines. Consultation provides a useful model for some aspects of tutoring, for example. The only problem is that reality often dictates that here the two forms of supervision, consultative and hierarchical, may overlap.

Concluding note

Consultation is particularly useful in training for learning about other people's roles and skills, whether when working in another part of the world, perhaps a very deprived area, or when working with a highly specialised team. It is a good general purpose method of finding out who does what.

Most of the examples here were 'set piece' activities designed for special teaching events, and had a lot in common with role play, team-building exercises and similar activities which are increasingly seen in professional training, though perhaps more outside the healthcare field than within it. However, my impression is that while such exercises can show participants what it feels like to be a client, or disabled, or a leader, or whatever, they can have something of the qualities of a beached sea creature: interesting at the time, but of lasting interest to only a handful of specialists once the crowds have drifted away. I suggest that the core concept of systems consultation (quite a hard core within a necessarily fuzzy exterior), is about working hard at finding out how the other person in the transaction perceives, thinks and feels, and has a role in making sense of a whole range of whole-system, whole-person training endeavours. In this sense the consultative approach is very close to being an applied science and art of self-management as well as management, and of empathy; it is an attitude and style of work, as well as a set of techniques.

CHAPTER 8

Consultation in assessing and managing clinical problems

- Combining clinical and systems consultation.
Examples:
- Consultative–diagnostic approaches in child psychiatry.
- Problematic diabetes in an adolescent.
- A disturbed child: treatment, care or control?

Introduction

As already pointed out, systems and similar consultative methods were originally developed to help professional workers work and train together, doing so by specific approaches which included mutual respect as equals and acknowledgement of each other's respective authority, skills and responsibilities, not attitudes which can be taken for granted in interdisciplinary relationships. (Later we will be exploring how this approach can be adapted to the relationships between healthcare workers and their clientele.)

The core idea is that professionals undertaking systems consultation should leave their own particular clinical skills behind them, the primary task being to help the *other* workers, the consultees, use theirs. However, I am proposing that a doctor or other therapist who is clear about his or her own clinical role and skills, and who knows about systems consultation skills, should be able to switch between one role and the other whenever this is likely to be useful. This proposition can meet resistance: thus a psychotherapist may see himself or herself as only and totally in a psychotherapeutic relationship with the client, anything outside this self-imposed discipline undermining the work. This is certainly one way of working; but another is I think in terms of what one does, as opposed to what one 'is', so that a psychotherapist or any other health worker can shift to a consultative mode when that is useful for some specific reason, and, as always in consultative work, the consultee understands the reason for the change.

In Example 11, I showed how this represented 'adapting' (more accurately, breaking) the rules, for example when someone was employed as a systems consultant but on commonsense grounds spotted a special need to help the consultees with a piece of clinical information. In this chapter, however, I will discuss combining clinical and systems consultation in a routine way.

Child and family psychiatry as a paradigm for systems work in healthcare

My interest in the systems model of assessment and treatment, and consultation as the means of applying it, resulted from attempts to make sense of what presented in child and adolescent psychiatry. Individual clinical diagnosis and individual treatment alone was almost always insufficient; on the other hand, the purely systems approach favoured by some family therapists left important things out.

To put the systems consultative approach into perspective in the context of clinical work, I think one should have a spectrum of response in mind (*see* Figure 17). At one end there will be occasions when the amount of consultation indicated or possible is zero, for example, when a medical worker comes across a patient in a state of acute collapse where not even informal consent can be sought. Another example would be intervening physically in a violent incident simply to make the situation safe where there is no immediate way of knowing why it is happening.

At the other end of the spectrum there are times when there is, in a healthcare sense, 'nothing' wrong, for example misunderstanding or lack of

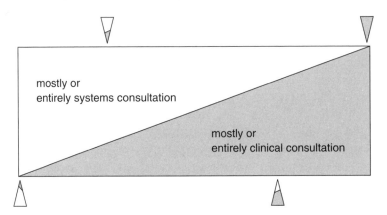

Figure 17:   At each point in the spectrum not *whether* systems or clinical consultantion, but *how much* of each.

knowledge about an aspect of development or behaviour in a child, or some kind of personal event, which requires only exploration and explanation.

The whole of medicine and healthcare generally can be placed at various points along this spectrum, and where to put each could be a lively subject for debate. However, speaking for child psychiatry I would say that it spans the whole spectrum, and Example 18 demonstrates this. It is rather contrived (like those illustrations in children's books which show *all* the denizens of the deep swimming about in the same place) but is at the same time authentic.

Example 18: consultative–diagnostic approaches in child psychiatry

A young woman of 23 brings her 7-year-old boy to see her family doctor. She is concerned that the child is hyperactive, and his school has asked if he could 'receive treatment' if he is to stay there. The doctor finds the child behaving quite reasonably in the surgery, but his mother seems very depressed, and while the child potters about the room (until hauled firmly onto her lap) she hints at a very troubled relationship with her new partner, who is not the child's father. The doctor suggests another appointment, without the child, but it is difficult for the woman to take more time off work *and* to ask her mother-in-law (one of the few people who can cope with him) to look after him. He prescribes antidepressants for her and asks his community nurse to visit her at home.

Before she can do so, a message from the local hospital informs the GP that the woman has been seen there for a minor overdose of drugs, and a message from the school reports that the boy has now been suspended, pending treatment, having attacked a younger child.

He sees the young woman again, and this time she comes armed with some papers a friend has given her: they are newspaper reports and Internet printouts about Attention Deficit Hyperkinetic Disorder (ADHD), incorporating the view that it is a diagnosis often missed, and that it can respond swiftly, indeed within hours, to stimulant medication like methylphenidate, with the child's behaviour being returned to normal.

The Child Psychiatric Clinic is able to see the child quickly. Two or three of the clinic staff (psychiatrist, psychologist, social worker) see the mother and child. They also ask if her new partner can come. He refuses. However, the boy's natural father and his own mother attend, with permission. The man, silent initially, then becomes enraged about any possibility of his son being 'drugged', and complains bitterly about the boy's mother's friend, a 'busybody' who had no business telling her to get the child put on medication. If any such plan goes ahead, he will take the whole matter back to court and ask for custody of the child.

Meanwhile, the school, whom the clinic has contacted, say that they have seen astonishingly good results with similar children from being prescribed methylphenidate, and that they have a teacher who particularly keeps an eye on such children and their medication. They hope this child will be similarly treated soon, because they are anxious for his return. Indeed, his class has sent a 'get well' card, signed by everybody, even the child who was assaulted.

The reports from home and school show typical symptoms of ADHD in the child, and they are worsening.

The clinic's assessment in liaison with the family doctor shows no physical illness behind the boy's symptoms and no reason why he should not have a trial of medication. Standardised questionnaires show that by these criteria the boy's problems are just about characteristic of ADHD – on the borderline. A management plan is drawn up which involves the clinic's social worker undertaking a family assessment as soon as she can (though when she is able to finally fix an appointment the woman's current partner goes and gets drunk). The psychologist will arrange with the school a behavioural regime to help manage the boy's behaviour, and similarly advise the family on systematic parenting skills, although it isn't clear who will actually be spending most time with the child. He gets on better with his natural father than with his mother's new partner. Nearly everyone is willing to give it a try, although the school is dismayed at how long the intervals must be between the busy psychologist's appointments, and cannot have the boy back unless quick and sustained progress can be assured. The boy's natural father warns that, first, his ex-wife's new partner will never play a helpful part in this programme, and second, he himself will take all steps necessary to prevent the child having medication, despite not having custody of the child.

The young woman herself is desperate to get back to her work, for the income and for the chance to be back with her friends and out of the house. Her partner is worse than ever, demanding and often drunk, and the young woman's ex-husband and his mother are saying 'I told you so' about him and threatening a return to court, attributing the little boy's behaviour to all the distress and upset in the reconstituted family. She pleads: 'Can't you just give the medication a *try?*'

The psychologist thinks that the team will just have to sweat it out and get a reasonable behaviour programme up and running first. The social worker thinks there should be no question of medication for the time being because the family disruption and distress is so obvious. Yet at the same time the little boy's behaviour patterns are characteristic of borderline ADHD. Meanwhile, the boy's natural father has faxed to the clinic several feet of printouts from newspapers and Internet information, detailing the evils of grossly inappropriate medication for so-called hyperactivity.

Comments

1 The example is contrived, though not much, and any child and family clinic will confirm that cases resembling this one present frequently. They are manageable (requiring the kind of time which makes child psychiatric clinic waiting lists long), and the following notes point out the strands in the various systems that have to be attended to.

2 ADHD exists and methylphenidate medication can work, and work very quickly; and, with manageable precautions, safely. This fact does not detract from the other issues (e.g. *see* Schachar and Ickowicz 2000).

3 ADHD is a puzzle. It is on a spectrum with the classical and well-researched symptoms of the syndrome at one end but merging with less well-defined conduct disorder at the other.

4 It is as certain as anything can be that the child's broken and reconstituted family and his mother's distress and depression are contributing to his problems.

   Even if this were not pretty certain, there is no doubt that individual and family help and consultation with the teachers will be needed to enable his handling at home and school to be back on an even keel; and the prospect of prescribing medication in a chaotic home situation gives pause for thought, quite apart from the child's natural father's opposition and threats. Quite complex negotiation is needed to identify and affirm who will actually be responsible for implementing a home behavioural programme, and thus whom to work with, bearing in mind that the young mother is dependent socially, emotionally and financially on her job, and her partner (whom she loves) is veering between being merely negative and quite destructive.

5 Her fondness for her new partner is real; but he has emotional and drug-dependency problems of his own. One of her many fears is that she will not be a 'good enough' mother, just as her mother-in-law and ex-husband say, and that he will be able to regain care and custody of the child. The reason for divorcing the boy's natural father was because of his violence towards her, but the little boy likes him and behaves better in his company. Thus the estranged part of the family has considerable informal power over her, and, conceivably, this could become backed by the court. Handling this side of this diffuse problem could be complicated, lengthy, and straddle medical, social and legal issues.

6 Meanwhile, the situation contains all sorts of pressures and urgencies: the woman's wish, or need, for a quick return to her job, which requires her son's swift return to school. She is still depressed, with suicidal thoughts.

7 In this well ordered clinic we can leave out conflict within the team about how best to proceed. But this does happen, and can cause problems in decision making just when clarity is needed.

8 ADHD is a real clinical entity with demonstrably effective treatment possible, usually combined family and behavioural work, closely monitored, to which medication is added if the social and psychological approaches prove insufficient. In textbook terms it is pretty straightforward. The other side of this, however, is the need to appreciate the complex system in which both child and clinician are embedded. It involves issues of consent, and determination of who can give this consent. Time is a factor, because the matter is urgent, but time is needed to enable changes in school and family behaviour to take effect; and time is important in another way, because a complete change in family circumstances (e.g. in care and custody) can't be ruled out. Moreover, progress is likely to be slow and erratic and open to different interpretations, unless medication is prescribed, if agreed and if it worked.

All this would need consultation with the school, with influential relatives and possibly at some stage with solicitors and court officers. Each clinical worker involved best proceeds two-handedly, with clinical skills on the one hand and consultative skills on the other, each set of skills finely tuned to the clinical problem but also to a wider, contextual muddle of feelings, roles and legal issues.

9 Finally, this account could be read as if sensible parents and a competent team could get on with helping the child if only all these other people weren't interfering so dramatically and constructively. But the estranged father could be 'right' in his opposition to medication, and the boy's natural mother 'right' in her ultimate hopes for her new partner. And these opinions may shift or change. Even scientific studies of the treatment of ADHD and the role of medication are likely to change from time to time.

The situation is complex and chaotic but represents issues common in child psychiatry and child care. Without being unduly alarmist I think they will be increasingly apparent in general medical and healthcare too: the undercurrents, certainly, are there in an increasing number of fields (Steinberg 2004b and page 58 *et seq*). But perhaps more importantly, I think many issues represented here in high relief are present less obviously in what one might call 'easier' cases involving more polite and deferential clients; they too deserve our attention.

Example 19: a consultative–diagnostic approach in adult psychiatry

For some relief, a shorter account. A young man diagnosed with schizophrenia is to be discharged from hospital to an after-care hostel. Proper management of his condition requires both careful monitoring of his fluctuating symptoms and his medication, and just as much care with the way he is worked with in the hostel. His parents would like him home in due course, and have already been involved with the family work that is now recommended and is (ideally) standard practice in the management of schizophrenia. The role of the clinical team is twofold, essentially seeking to clarify, in consultation with patient, hostel and family: what can we contribute, as clinicians? And what can the hostel and the young man's family contribute?

Comment

The issues described in the previous example might have their counterparts in this situation too. Conversely, the relatively simple formula What can we do? What can you do? What can someone else do? is a good way to begin to find one's way into even the most complex and hair-raising of healthcare situations. But it requires negotiation, not simple 'questions and answers', and that is systems consultation.

Example 20: consultative–diagnostic approach in general medicine

A teenage girl with diabetes is admitted with an overdose of tranquillisers and analgesics. A careful history shows that her recent history of unstable diabetes is likely to have the same basic causes as her overdose: a marital crisis between her parents, depression, deteriorating friendships and school performance, and self-neglect. Psychiatric and general medical 'first aid' appears to patch up her depression, the management of her diabetes and (using the 'who is in the best position to do what?' formula (Example 19)) the physician and a social work colleague help the family in the process of coming together again. They encourage a teacher the girl likes to have a special role in her pastoral care at school, and establish a diabetic treatment schedule, overseen by the general practice nurse, which the girl undertakes to follow. But she still mismanages her diabetes, despite the best of apparent intentions and things seeming better at home and at school. Matters are explored again; several key things appear genuinely improved, but refocusing on the girl's individual feelings and motivation reveals a bitterness about having diabetes and being dependent on adults and having to be careful about her diet ever since the beginning of her adolescence. She does not now want to harm herself, and is enjoying the new situation at school, but her feelings about her condition are still fuelling a degree of self-neglect and carelessness. She is seen by a nurse with counselling training for a number of therapeutic sessions focusing on how her diabetes affects her sense of independence and autonomy.

Again, she makes real progress, and while she is doing so the nurse discusses with her supervisor the particular issue of whether a short series of sessions will be enough or whether formal psychotherapy might be needed at some point. However, something new emerges from consultation about this with the supervisor: it emerges that the girl has never before dared say that she fears going blind, like her diabetic grandmother. Despite her intelligence and general understanding of diabetes, her fears have stopped her thinking rationally about this aspect of her long-term care and outlook. A move from a primarily therapeutic approach to a primarily educational one, which the nurse is well qualified to undertake, brings about a lasting improvement.

Comment

What I have tried to illustrate here is another aspect of the systemic approach, that it can pursue changes happening on a broad front. People and their disorders shift and change with time, with new developments, and with shifts of treatment and the results of treatment. Here, doctor and nurse-counsellor have followed a consultative–diagnostic approach that dealt at successive stages with what clinicians can do, what others (parents, schoolteacher) can do, and what the girl herself can do; and then, with sensitivity and good timing (and following the regular consultation with a colleague which was part of the nurse counsellor's timetable), the counsellor changed tack from a therapeutic role to an educational one.

Example 21: behaviour disorder in a children's home: treatment or care and control?

Late on a Friday afternoon a psychiatrist is asked to urgently see a boy newly admitted to a children's home and acting aggressively without obvious reason. He has had to be brought back twice, having run off. The staff, who sound quite anxious, describe his 'glazed expression' and think he has 'something wrong' with him – perhaps epilepsy, perhaps mental illness – and they ask if he can be admitted right away to the young people's psychiatric unit for observation. The psychiatrist questions the caller closely and is satisfied that the boy is showing signs neither of epilepsy nor of psychiatric illness but is reacting to his sudden admission from an acutely broken down home situation, and that with a mixture of setting limits plus 'tender loving care' he should settle down.

He does, that evening. But the next morning the psychiatrist finds that the boy has been admitted overnight to his unit, having run away again. He had nearly been knocked down by a car (apparently an accident, but the staff aren't sure), been taken to the Accident Department, and then admitted 'overnight' because the children's home staff said they could not take further responsibility for him. The night staff, it seems, are threatening to leave. Asking about the boy's social worker's view of this development, he is told that a message for her was left with the Social Services Duty Officer in the early hours and that she will no doubt be in touch.

Comments

1 The psychiatrist had taken the view, having questioned the staff member about key symptoms and signs, that the boy was not unwell, did not need to be seen at the hospital, and was clearly in the right place – the children's home.
2 Instead, once (quite quickly) establishing these things, he could have widened his questions to ask not only what seemed to be troubling the boy, but what seemed to be troubling the staff. He would have found that the two staff on that night were relatively new, and one was 'acting up' for a senior person who was off sick. Further, that the children's home had been criticised recently for its residents' high rate of absconding and getting into trouble. The psychiatrist was right to take a diagnostic line with some of his questions, but consultative questions about the kind of system the child had come into (its recent history, its staffing) and their skills – how they usually handled children in this boy's situation – might have helped the staff cope, especially if a provisional observation and management plan using their skills had been put together. This would have taken a little longer, but not so long as it could take to get the child back to this or another home; and meanwhile the child has had two further moves (in and then in due course out of hospital) to add to the trauma of removal from home.
3 The child's social worker is not happy about the 'emergency' and would have wanted to be involved in a crisis meeting with the children's home staff about their problems with him. When she had left the boy there the day staff were on duty, and all seemed well. Overall, the situation, with a young person in a hospital where he does not need to be, and with no obvious home to go to, has become a mess. Systemic consultation about what the children's home was like rather than simply what the child was like might have avoided this. In children's cases it is important to explore care and control issues, whether or not a clinical diagnosis exists and some form of treatment is needed (Steinberg 1981, 1982, 1983, 1987; Steinberg et al. 1981), and the key people must include whoever has formal responsibility for the child, which will be the parents, social worker or an appointed guardian. There are many cases of problem behaviour in boys and girls where proper and sustained care and control makes 'treatment' unnecessary, and it is

systems consultation that can determine who is in a position to do what in these respects.

Concluding note

Clinical enquiry is so well established that it has been necessary to distinguish systems consultation from it, to show how broader considerations than the strictly clinical may be taken into account too. Doctors have long been taught to take a 'family history' and a 'social history' along with the clinical history, but this tends to be cursory, with highly complex matters (like 'occupation', 'marital status' or 'religion') being reduced to little more information than might appear on the front sheet of the notes. The consultative approach takes the whole of healthcare, including the skills, perspectives and attitudes of our colleagues, the organisations where we work *and* the whole of patients' lives, as every bit as complex as the anatomical and physiological lengths and depths that clinical enquiry covers, and is fully complementary to it. I hope it could be seen that taking a combined consultative and diagnostic approach in healthcare is like applying binocular vision.

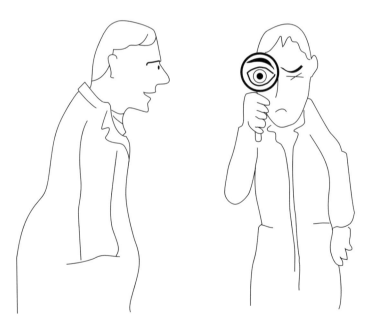

Figure 18: 'Can you try opening the other eye?'.

CHAPTER 9

Consultation as self-management: consulting with oneself

- The several sources of wisdom.
- How to proceed: the short, rough guide.
- An example: anorexia nervosa with complications.
- Making decisions in difficult circumstances.
- The consultative components of self-management.

Remembrance of things past

Faced with a problem large or small whose resolution isn't immediately obvious, and where there is unlikely to be a textbook answer to recall or look up, we tend to use a combination of our own knowledge and experience plus, sometimes, the recollection of what X or Y would have done. He or she might be an experienced colleague, past or present, and sometimes a teacher who made an impression. One of my own teachers, comparing the beautifully typed notes of one colleague who had given an opinion on a patient, with the ballpen scrawl of another, advised us to take care not to give the nicely presented stuff more credence: 'Just because it's nicely typed doesn't mean it's true'.

The message was something about always going back to the first principles of enquiry, even somewhat sceptically, a sine qua non in scientific enquiry and evident also in the best clinical teaching: a patient says he has a pain in his chest; what does he mean by pain, exactly? And where does he mean, by 'chest'? This kind of thing was a factor in my interest in the consultative style of enquiry, which was also about not relying on preconceived assumptions about complex matters and the pulling-out of familiar solutions, but on questioning everything. The clinical tradition has largely continued in much the same way; but there is a tendency towards the wider aspects of enquiry, into what I have called the 'other', more psychosocial, side of medicine, becoming formulated into, say, a psychodynamic model of explanation being favoured in one institution, a family model somewhere else, and everywhere an increasing acreage of recommendations, protocols, checklists and guidelines produced by big science and big administration.

I think the basic questions that clinical methods teach us equip the clinician, wherever he or she goes, with or without books, with or without colleagues, at least for most diagnoses, if not for treatment. I think the systematic questioning of clinical work has its parallels in consultation, although in the latter one is tracking a number of very different systems. Given this mode of enquiry, stuck with a problem without a colleague at hand with whom to consult, it can be a helpful start to think through not so much 'what would X have done here?' but 'what would X have wanted to know?' Or indeed, if you have had some experience of consultation, what would *you* have wanted to know, as consultant, as consultee, or both?

The first requirement is a relatively calm frame of mind, which one hopes would be recollected in a friendly and supportive (if searching) consultative session where one can stand back from the problem. Perhaps the practitioner could have one of those collapsible wood-and-canvas chairs available, labelled not 'Director' but 'Consultant', to move to from the hot seat when under pressure. I am not entirely serious about that, but the mental picture of some such move would be useful. A time-creating strategy is also useful; the rushed, frantic patient or colleague in a hurry for an answer might have all sorts of unconscious reasons to see *you* jolted into being rushed and frantic too, but he or she will in fact appreciate and respect a cooler response, and if necessary the request for a few quiet moments to think.

I have the impression that sometimes even thinking of something that worked before can help now, sometimes instantly. Having spent some time training in relaxation techniques (imagery, breathing exercises and similar things) I have found, between patients and phone calls in hectic clinics, that even a few seconds simply recalling their existence was remarkably cooling; something worth researching, I think, and reminding me of a distinguished pharmacologist who told me that the moment he took an aspirin he was able to devote his mind to other things than his headache; the tablet was working before it had even been swallowed.

Remember also the lessons of situations like that described on page 83. Ability to cope is not only a matter of personality, experience and reflection, but having the tools for the job in terms of space, equipment and a time-table that isn't too obviously crazy.

The kinds of question to ask about complex situations: a summary

1   Who, exactly, is complaining about what?
2   Are all the people with the necessary information, authority and respon-sibility available and, if necessary, involved?
3   The traditional question – what, then, seems to be the trouble?
4   Who is in a position to help? How?
5   In due course – how is it going so far?

Example 22: anorexia nervosa, in a boarding school

Who is complaining about what?

A teenage girl in a residential school is referred to a child psychiatric clinic because treatment of her anorexia nervosa isn't working. The school nurse, advised by the school doctor, has advised her firmly about her weight loss, and has her on a planned diet monitored by regular weighing. The Head has now warned her that if she doesn't make progress she may have to leave the school, which has had problems with intractable anorexia nervosa before.

• The Head is concerned about the girl's anorexia nervosa, and the school as a whole.
• The nurse is concerned that her treatment isn't working.
• The girl says that nothing is wrong, and she doesn't know what all the fuss is about. She says her father agrees with her.

Are the people with the necessary information, authority and responsibility involved?

Clearly not. Thus far the girl's parents are out of the picture, even though the nurse confirms that the Head has parents' automatic permission to refer children for medical advice as necessary. This policy is because many of the parents at the school are often busy elsewhere; the girl's mother is an inter-national journalist and the father a civil engineer. The clinic asks for parental agreement to the referral and for both parents to attend the clinic.

Why? Because as well as the internal psychophysiological causes of anorexia nervosa there is evidence that in many cases external systems at home and in school play a part too.

- The Head appreciates this and offers the girl's personal tutor and the nurse as people who can take part in close liaison with the clinic. This is an excellent idea, but it also emerges that –
- while the girl's mother is profoundly anxious about her daughter's anorexia (she was once severely anorexic herself and knows how bad it can be), the girl's father agrees with the girl: 'it is a lot of fuss about nothing'; further, he doesn't like the school or its Head and thinks his daughter should change schools, which is a source of constant turbulence between the parents, especially as exams (which the girl fears, being over-conscientious and obsessional) are coming up.
- The daughter meanwhile misses both parents but agrees with her father (a) that there is nothing wrong with her, (b) that she hates the school and would like to change.

What seems to be the trouble?

- Clinical enquiry reveals the characteristic symptoms and signs of anorexia nervosa, including a phobia of gaining weight and denial that it is a problem.
- Few patients with anorexia are helped by the inevitably slow process of individual psychotherapy. The necessary personal change is more likely to be achieved by establishing trusted external authority at the earliest opportunity, not as the primary treatment but as a precondition for it. However, father, mother and Head have rather different concerns and agendas. The parents and the Head need to re-establish more consistent, precise rules and roles, acknowledging that whatever the Head's natural concern for the girl, what matters is that she is insisting that something changes. The parents can't have it both ways (i.e. saying the problem is/ isn't important, and that the girl should/needn't stay at the school) or rather, they can, but this confusion about who wants what feeds into the girl's need to gain *some* sort of feeling of control in a distressing situation, which she has done by gaining phobic-obsessive control of her weight. That's one thing in her life that *does* work. Thus answering this question requires a clinical hypothesis for what may be happening within the girl and a systemic model for what may be happening without.

    Thus the problems are

    (i)   lack of progress in clinical treatment
    (ii) different views about treatment on the parents' parts

(iii) no wish for treatment on the prospective patients' part

(iv) the Heads reluctance to have an unwell girl on the roll.

- With regard to treatment so far by school doctor and nurse, anorexia nervosa can be hard to treat, and there is evidence that patients do better with the most experienced teams, just as one might expect with, say, specialised surgery.

  To take other examples, diabetic patients may misunderstand or (as some troubled teenagers do – as in Example 20) even sabotage their treatment. Drugs prescribed may not be prescribed in sufficient doses or for long enough, or patients may not take them regularly or at all. A common finding in child psychiatry is that the night alarm for enuresis (a very effective treatment) is either not being used properly (e.g. with dying batteries) or not for long enough. In the present type of case, by no means uncommon, the school nurse was very competent at managing the practicalities of anorexia nervosa but was *also* trying to combine this role with being an individual and sympathetic counsellor to the girl (including being drawn into haggling about whether a particular weight gain was sufficient or not) and trying to use her authority as school nurse to insist on treatment. But real authority in this girl's case rested with the Head and the two parents, all with different needs and perspectives. Thus *authority* was divided between Head and two parents, but *responsibility* was with the nurse.

  As far as the girl's own authority and consent go, there are yet more grey areas. The simple rule is that at age 16 a child is able to give (or withhold) consent for treatment themselves. But with somewhat older children, parents can in certain (medically serious) circumstances have their views taken into account too; while in some situations to do with sexuality younger children can act autonomously, here the issue of consent (and confidentiality) depends on the level of understanding, maturity and competence to make reasonable decisions. All this is fraught with complexity, ambiguity and uncertainty and is part of the burgeoning volume of issues where individual doctors and their colleagues are expected (or expect themselves) to have a definite position while the most experienced lawyers, scientists and philosophers might not.

Who is in a position to do what, to help the girl?

The role of the Head however is to lay down the law about what degree of illness or disability is compatible with the school curriculum. The role of the parents is to obtain and authorise treatment for their child and to meet the requirements of the school.

What was needed was the *Head's* authority to insist that the *parents* reached a decision about treatment if their daughter was to remain at the school. Consultation clarified this and also that the parents could not assume that all would be well with this life-threatening disorder if she simply changed schools – if that step was possible in her present state. Staying at the school required adherence to the school doctor's and nurse's treatment programme, and evidence of weight gain. The consultant's role here was to stand back and remind all concerned of their respective roles, authority and responsibility; and this included exploring the girl's wish or need for individual psychological therapy or for an advocate of her own.

Finally: how is it all going?

The various above aims constitute a kind of job card for all concerned, including the girl and parents, and form the basis for monitoring progress in some way, in this case through charting weight and health, the family meetings and occasional meetings with the school staff. This kind of negotiated and planned programme of clinical, clinical-consultative and consultative sessions is likely to be less time-consuming than ad hoc attempts at managing different parts of a fluctuating and complex problem, and certainly less costly than hospital admission. Allotting different tasks to the different people involved, and holding meetings to review progress, again reminds everyone of their responsibilities and authority.

Comment

Psychiatry lends itself to this sort of systems and clinical analysis because the findings are the stuff not only of aetiology, but are preconditions of proper management. Indeed, one can hardly separate that which helps cause a problem and that which is needed to unravel it, again evidence of the validity of the systems rather than the linear model of understanding disorder. It is helpful to have a simple 'clinical-consultative' system in the back of one's mind to work out who's seeking to do what for or to whom, and with what authority and consistency. Also as pointed out, the healthcare practitioner versed in such approaches no more needs a vast psycho-socio-organisational bible to refer to than the clinician needs to have every page of *Gray's Anatomy* at hand. What matters is a general awareness of what else may be relevant: a kind of healthcare road sense. The reasonably calm detachment the clinician needs is more likely to be undermined by these grey matters and fuzzy issues than by severity of symptons. The advice is to have 'grey anatomy' in mind alongside *Gray*.

What is it like, being a clinician?

People entering the healthcare field from any perspective are likely to find the following: an overwhelming and constantly expanding body of knowledge whose basic principles are in a dozen or more basic sciences; a huge penumbra of additional organisational and inter-professional factors – those outlined in this book; ambiguities, dilemmas and controversies (academic as well as in terms of public opinion) which – to repeat the comparison – even a High Court calling endless witnesses or a month-long conference could never resolve to everyone's, or even most people's, satisfaction; a tendency to organisational complexity and inefficient use of every kind of resource (including each practitioner's time); and a high level of demand, physically, intellectually and emotionally, which leaves people tired.

Within this matrix of uncertainty the doctor and those in all healthcare who aspire to work like doctors have to make decisions, sometimes very urgent ones. Having to 'act amidst ambiguity' was how Eisenberg (1975) identified the dilemma.

In other words, the job, or at least the job description as above, is impossible. Now impossible jobs are manageable if the extreme difficulty is acknowledged, but it tends not to be, because many people drawn to healthcare tend to have a strong streak of wanting to help and rescue people, a need to seem in control, plus more than a fair share of conscientiousness, among many other quite different motivations, and this of course is what their clientele want them to have too. The client wants the magic of total understanding and a reliable and not too painful cure; the doctor tends to want, or need, total charge. Both expectations are impossible, and in general we get by with variable degrees of gratitude and disappointment. A common undercurrent in the clinical relationship is the transaction where one participant, the clinician, is accorded great respect, as long as he or she will take over, take the pain away and perform magic. It is a powerful collusion, liable to lead to disappointment.

Do we like our patients? Does it matter? 'Liking', or 'inter-personal attraction' has been identified as a key factor in the doctor–patient relationship (e.g. Lings *et al.* 2003), and how much the doctor liked the patient has been found to correlate positively with both the doctor's and the patient's satisfaction (Like and Zyzanski 1987). In this context Kubacki (2003) raises the question of whether liking equates with rapport, which I think is not necessarily so. A good rapport, I think, is a good working relationship, and might apply as much in, for example, good mutual understanding about the pros and cons of a surgical operation and the difficulties of making a decision, as in work between a psychiatrist and a schizophrenic patient. In these two examples the nature of 'liking' would probably be different, and yet whatever it amounted to, perhaps feelings of trust and positive regard, would have to underpin something intuitive on the one hand and cognitive on the other to take it a step nearer 'rapport'.

And what about the clinician's dislike of patients, and vice versa? Working in hospitals I am often surprised at the number of patients complaining bitterly about the personality and style of their family doctors or other specialists, yet with no intent or even interest in changing them; conversely, as a reader of what might be called the 'popular' magazines written by and for doctors, one can only assume that the spleen often vented about patients by correspondents and columnists is effectively cathartic, and results in more kindly exchanges in the consulting room.

Such considerations, plus the pressure from without and within to do the right thing swiftly, can make it difficult to think through the kinds of complexity discussed in this book, and highlighted in this chapter.

Of course, where particular problems and crises are familiar and acknowledged, clear procedures are established and taught. What to do, for example, for a patient with cardiac arrest, or the catastrophic damage of a traffic accident or a bomb, or an acute, severe allergic reaction. But most of medical care isn't like this, and for that 80 or 90%, in which I include the themes chosen for this book, there is rather little teaching or systematic guidance, and regular supervision, or tutoring, or mentoring, is relatively uncommon. The lack of explicit recognition of how to handle impossible problems, indeed acknowledgement that they *are* impossible, is particularly noticeable in medicine and much of nursing too, while psychotherapy and counselling it is practically routine. All jobs have their pressures, and it is noticeable that tough-minded organisations like the armed forces, the police and industry seem to have shown more interest over a longer period in the supposedly 'softer' psychology of particular kinds of occupation and activity, and in providing specialist training and care for their personnel in these respects, than have the health services. Even so, while the former fields of work expect trouble, many problems in the healthcare field seem self-inflicted and unnecessary. All of this is antithetical to a field keeping its most important tools – its staff – in good shape.

Consulting with oneself as self-management

A reminder about the core purpose of consultation: it provides a setting (one-to-one or in a group) which is deliberately arranged so that the people involved can stand back from the task in which they may have become 'nose-to-nose', put things into perspective, and in a cooler frame of mind take time to consider all the necessary factors involved in the nature of the matter in hand, and what to do about it. The notion of 'consulting with oneself' means that given the experience of analysing problems into their multiple constituent systems with the help of another person, it can become part of one's professional repertoire to think through tricky matters by asking oneself: where would systems consultation lead me in this? And people who have been involved in consultation teaching and learning report that this is in fact what happens. Consulting with oneself becomes second nature, and is part of the self-management which should be integral to managing an office, a practice, a team, a unit or a department.

To pick out a few components of this process:

1 In the example with which this chapter began, any of the people mentioned (teacher, nurse, doctor, the Head, a member of the psychiatric clinic team) may be involved in a broadly similar case at some time in the future, perhaps about another kind of problem entirely. The way of thinking through the types of questions listed on page 131 can be recalled, and often is, as an experience, or skill, reasonably identified as consulting with oneself. It may still leave left-over problems, but these will now have become highlighted, the ground cleared so to speak, and can become a sharpened focus for brief consultation with someone else. Either way, the problem-clarifying, problem-solving skills will now be part of the healthcare worker's experience and repertoire.

2 Having a way of managing the apparently or potentially unmanageable returns autonomy to the practitioner. He or she may not be in 'total control', but will be able to sift out what he or she should take charge of, and what someone else should take charge of, which represents reasonable control rather than chaos, tension, feelings of helplessness and consequent guilt. The chapter opened with some thoughts about how the decks might be cleared to make space, time and energy for this.

3 That much applies to particular events; but it should inform the healthcare worker's whole work ethic, life style and philosophy. There is a choice between being a workaholic heading for maximum achievement or burnout, and being a competent practitioner with enough enjoyment

of the job to have time, energy, empathy, generosity and imagination left over for the clientele, for colleagues and for trainees. What individuals should do to maintain their own health, strength, happiness and sense of proportion is for each to decide, though my impression is that sometimes particular activities are pursued outside work to make work tolerable rather than enjoyable, which I think is something that should be everyone's right to expect. There are some thoughts about this in Chapters 11 and 12.

4   Dealing with feelings: Strong feelings and attitudes emerge in working relationships with colleagues and with clients. Feelings of worry, sadness and anger about colleagues and patients may be entirely appropriate, whether or not there are also personal difficulties which have become autonomous rather than work-related. An issue in the clinician–consultant's reflection about an emotive matter is how much of all this is for private resolution, with or without outside help, and how much is work-focused and part of the task for consultation. As pointed out earlier, it is a consultation skill to allow for the degree of upset that work-related issues and work-related relationships can cause, and to assume the consultee's 'self-righting' capacity, however much buffeted about, once something is being done about the cause of the turbulence. This kind of issue is important, not only when something peaks as a crisis, but in the routine minor ups and down of work too.

   For some the experience of reflection with colleagues helps both at the time *and* when recollected, whether in the form of supervision, mentoring, consultation (e.g. team reflection: *see* Sluzki 1999) or approaching the sources of advice now available through professional bodies. Consulting with any of these is likely to be helpful, and this experience too may help the reflective process of consulting with oneself.

5   And finally, on the well-intentioned but uncertain nature of 'support'; the word sounds a little like an emotional version of a truss to me, or diluted psychotherapy. I think the best support is good training, regular in-service supervision or consultation of some sort, and the ability to take confident pleasure in one's work. To this I would add the space, time and occasions to reflect about the nature of the job, *and acceptance that constant turbulence is part of it*. This combination of the technical and clinical skills for the nucleus of the work, plus discovering through systems consultation about its penumbra – its other side – should form the core of a rewarding system of training in healthcare: rewarding for clinicians, our colleagues and our clientele. When this penumbra becomes something capable of being understood and handled, instead of something irritating and peripheral in one's field of vision and understanding, it can become not merely manageable but

interesting. This too is a key move in consultation: shifting the frame and focus to wherever the problem really is, rather than staying stuck with preconceptions and assumptions about what the problem is supposed to be.

CHAPTER 10

Consulting the client: the patient as specialist

- From peer–peer consultation to doctor–patient relationships.
- A pause for thought about a cause: patient autonomy.
- Systems consultation as a model for doctor–patient collaboration.
- Letter writing.

Introduction

This chapter will briefly review some of the recent developments in the idea that has come to be called 'patient empowerment'. The phrase contains the feel of confrontation, and as I have pointed out, particularly in the next chapter, words carry with them some seeds of meaning not always consciously intended by their users. Is it confrontation that is wanted? Or needed? Meanwhile, 'patient empowerment' is a good banner with which to rally the huge literature on doctors and other clinicians and therapists as 'the baddies'. In this chapter I suggest a different approach, not because it is a 'middle way' or an easier option (it is neither) but because I believe it is likely to be more effective.

In essence, if the consultative approaches so far described enabled constructive, peer–peer dialogues between one professional specialist and another, not despite their different positions and perspectives *but because of* their different positions and perspectives, and *explicitly* focusing on, valuing and putting to use their different perceptions, why not see if the same consultative dialogue can be used to inform the doctor–patient or therapist–client relationship?

Anderson (1995) has used in this context what she describes in terms of a postmodernist perspective because of its challenge to a whole range of fixed assumptions. These include knowledge and the possessor of knowledge as being independent of each other, or for language and phrases having fixed meanings in respect of that body of knowledge. She proposes conversations that acknowledge the fluidity of the concepts that we pretend are rock solid (like illness, diagnosis or treatment) and favours the construction of understanding from discussion. She argues for therapy as well as organisational consultation being a process of mutual enquiry which uses 'the clients' expertise on themselves, and the therapist's expertise on a process' (Anderson and Burney 1999; Anderson 1995, 1997). Deconstructionist 'postmodern' thinking is supposedly radical and new, although the assumptions of the nineteenth century have been challenged for at least 100 years by Freudian psychoanalysis and our intellectual developments. However, the many uncertainties in medicine and healthcare (e.g. the role of the intuitive) have tended to be set to one side in the pursuit of 'scientific' respectability and authority, particularly – as may be expected – in psychology and psychiatry, which, particularly in their mainstreams, have a need to render the immeasurable measurable at all costs.

Nevertheless, taken as a whole, medicine and quite a lot of psychology and psychiatry, mainstream, dissenting and radical, *has* come up with a whole array of useful facts and perspectives and effective treatments, so much so that keeping up to date with developments is a full-time job for the professional worker. Does this mean that if 'peer–peer' consultation between the hopeful patient and the knowledgeable clinician is encouraged, or undertaken, it is a one-sided exercise? I think it is not. My own interpretation of the core elements of the consultative task ('what is wanted, what is needed and what is possible'), and I think consistent with Anderson's position, is the idea of collaboration between the therapist as an authority on disorder and treatment in general, and the clients as authorities on themselves; although here I would make use of the double meaning in the word 'authority' to encapsulate both the clients' right to question and to decide, *and* their knowledge – that is, the information they have about themselves, their families and their own views on treatment in general, as well as their experience of their own disorder.

Consultation is not an intellectual exercise about reaching useful and usable therapeutic conclusions. In psychiatry in general, and child and adolescent psychiatry in particular (powerful learning areas because patients and their families are often less submissive and treatment approaches more controversial than in general medicine), getting informed consent is not just a matter of signing on the dotted line, a mere preliminary, but a serious and time-consuming first step in treatment and often an absolute precondition for it, whether the task is getting an anorexic teenager to keep appointments, keeping a suicidal patient in hospital or maintaining a patient's motivation and participation in psychotherapy (Steinberg 1987, 1989a, 1992; and *see* 2004b).

For all this, it is not that simple. The archetypal clinical relationship is very powerful. In the last chapter I referred to a kind of collusion between the very far from omniscient doctor and the apprehensive patient, in which the latter attributes magical powers to the former in return for recovery. A sceptic might point out that the other extreme is true – that patients tend not to trust doctors ('they never tell you anything') and expect wrong treatment at every turn. Of course, both extremes are true, and hence the potency of ambivalence.

To the psychiatrist such extremes aren't surprising, each being born out of the other, because when fantasy expectations come down to earth they do so with a damaging crash. Hence the bitterness, blame and litigation when things go wrong. The ideal, mature professional relationship would be based on rational expectations on both sides, but it would still be built on wobbly foundations, because when engaged in therapy there is trust in good fortune on both sides too, and even the most rational of patients hopes for some kind of a miracle when the outlook is bleak.

There are other reasons, too, why 'power sharing', to continue the political idiom, is not that easy to implement, with even the best of intentions, as shown by some of the work reviewed below.

Patient control of treatment

With a complex background that involves burgeoning information and misinformation, individual personalities and anxieties, everyone's rights and responsibilities, and ambiguities everywhere, it is not surprising that the debate about patient control of his or her treatment (e.g. Spiers 2003; Coulter 2003) between those generally inclined to be 'for' and those 'against' has not been entirely clear-cut.

Salmon and Hall (2004), for example, point out that while patient autonomy ought to be acceptable in every way – ethically, politically, and because of the evidence that gaining control over illness improves the ability to cope with it (e.g. Guadagnoli and Ward, 1998) – attempts to introduce it have been full of contradictions and ambiguities. Exercises in patient empowerment, defined in terms of 'letting patients choose the nature and timing of interventions' were full of unexpected difficulties, sometimes having only transient apparent benefits, and sometimes seeming even to favour *lack* of choice; for example, when the same authors found that patients allowed to control their own analgesic infusion tended to *underuse* it, presumably through apprehension, caution and misunderstanding, and consequently suffered more pain than necessary (Salmon and Hall 2001).

What was disconcerting in another kind of way was their discovery that 'patient compliance' (or submissiveness) extended even to 'patient empower-ment' itself – that patients taking over their own care was accepted as a policy 'if you think so, Doctor'. Thus there is a paradox in *imposing* patient empowerment, as it continues the tradition of 'Doctor (or nurse) knows best'.

An even darker side to patient empowerment is reported by the same authors where a child patient pleaded with apparently reluctant nurses to be allowed more time for the *self-administered* analgesic to work before being lifted and turned in bed. Presumably that aspect of patient empowerment was left out of the analgesia programme.

Overall these studies conclude that while patient empowerment sounds good in principle, more studies need to be undertaken on the emotional factors that 'are known to degrade clinician's relationships with patients (and which) help them to distance themselves psychologically from patients and to evade feelings of responsibility for the patient's pain and suffering' (Byrne *et al.* 2001). These and similar studies raise the question whether the supposed transfer of control for treatment to patients might actually be a transfer of responsibility rather than authority. In the words of Salmon and Hall (2001) 'when doctors, nurses and managers implement patient empowerment, or use the language of empowerment, they are taking part in redrawing the boundaries of medical responsibility'. I would emphasise the reference to 'the language of empowerment' here; saying something isn't the same as doing something, but we live in an age where the import-ance of the image is overtaking the importance of reality, hence Baudril-lard's words, 'the map is not the territory', at the beginning of this book. It is also a reminder of the work on hospitals by Menzies (1970), in which organisations can be shown to work steadily and systematically against their stated and no doubt believed aims.

Other studies which are neutral or negative about patient empowerment include those of Auerbach (2001), who found little evidence of patients seeking control of their clinical care, and Waterworth and Luker (1990), who found that they didn't want to be involved collaboratively. Possibly these apparently disappointing studies paradoxically represent good news: patients aren't being taken in. They probably suspect that our hearts aren't in it, and medical care is too complicated, particularly in emotional terms, for we in healthcare to believe that saying 'OK, you have a go then' guaran-tees genuine patient participation in choice and control. The problem, to me, is reminiscent of the push towards both-sex wards of some 20 years ago. Our ideological elite insisted it was the sensible and popular thing, indeed that it was old-fashioned, illiberal and even eccentric to doubt the wisdom and humanity of this step; since then, the mood of the ever-experimental elite has shifted, as it does, and the push is back in the other direction.

In the United Kingdom the government has now been adding patient choice to its many targets for health service improvements, but both strategies (for choice and for targets) nonetheless seem expert-led from the centre of power, the familiar governmental approach. Spiers (2003) has proposed that the only way adequately to put patients in charge of healthcare resources is by a radical restructuring of healthcare funding, involving a combination of compulsory insurance from competing providers offering legally enforceable contracts, funded by taxation and operated through a voucher system. In this way every patient would be able to purchase essential services, thereby still meeting the widely accepted criterion of service being 'free at the point of delivery', although people could also top up the basic package. Spiers suggests that there could be financial incentives to adopt healthy lifestyles, that prompt access to a core package of quality care would be guaranteed, and that there would be initiatives to take account of patients' preferences. Coulter (2003) has criticised this on the grounds that only basic care would be provided under this system and the rich would always be able to purchase better care, and – more to the point, I think – that although Spiers tries to circumvent services being rationed according to standardised needs assessments, nevertheless this is exactly what, between them, the government and the insurance providers would be doing. But in my view the core problem remains that medical provision and use remains complex and ambiguous *whoever* is paying and however they pay. It is not obvious – although it seems sometimes to be taken for granted by the critics of private healthcare – that when a prosperous man or woman seeks private care they get what *is* in fact the best and most appropriate for their needs. The issue, and of course the theme of this book, is that it is what happens *at the point of contact between clinician, clinician's colleagues and patient* that decides most about the nature and quality of care, for good or ill – whoever picks up the bill.

What is needed is not doctor–patient collaboration because it sounds good and reads well, or looks good in a 'customer-oriented' hospital brochure, or because it satisfies an ideological position, but attention to the actual *working process* of making doctor–patient collaboration a practical, teachable reality. Perhaps the ultimate test of patient empowerment, and a litmus test of the consultative exercise in exploring wants, needs and possibilities, would be the patient's right to have his or her wish fulfilled even should the wish defy prevailing convention: for example, to be treated as sick, tucked up in bed and told autocratically what to do. Another problem is that what we want (whether as patients or as professional workers) we may not always want all of the time, especially if we're not feeling well.

The question, then, is can the general principles of consultative work, designed for peer–peer collaboration between professionals, enable the clinician as expert to negotiate usefully with the client as expert, achieving the greatest good on the greatest number of issues? And can it do so sufficiently flexibly?

Inter-professional consultation applied to clinician and client

Would it be useful if the tripartite consultative question '*What is wanted, what is needed and what is possible?*' was as much second nature to the clinician and client as the clinical question '*What seems to be wrong?*' If this were a good idea, so that skill in consultation and public education went hand-in-hand with clinical knowledge (with which the broadcast and published media are already generous) it would encourage problem-handling strategies in those using health services, rather than as a policy imposed from outside. Its emergence and development would be educational, not administered; it could be taught at school.

The counter-argument that we *still* won't know if, or which, patients would want this approach to be introduced really doesn't matter. Because if pursued with logic and integrity, '*what is wanted*' could as already said lead to a preference for the clinician to decide (e.g. *see* Beaver *et al.* 1996) as much as to patient control; or negotiation about a position between the two. Thus the introduction, presumably through undergraduate and postgraduate training, of consultative skills that go beyond clinical consultation alone could introduce choice about control as one of the issues in the clinical relationship, rather than as an externally imposed grand plan. As to introducing the idea into the public domain, as a kind of 'how to get the best out of your doctor' kit: the notion is already there, but, as with so many good ideas, it is all over the place, inchoate and without its own terms and leverage. How could inter-professional consultation (referred to below as 'IPC'), with its own rules, style and a particular kind of mutuality in the consultant–consultee relationship, be adapted for professional–client use in healthcare?

IPC as a peer–peer activity

Any controversy about the notion that doctors might treat patients as peers is as nothing compared with the sparks that would fly if (as it must be put) *some* physicians, surgeons, academics, nurses, social workers, psychiatrists and other specialists, clinical psychologists, educational psychologists, teachers, hospital managers and many others involved in health and care were expected to treat others on this list as their equals. When I suggested as much about the field I knew best, child and adolescent psychiatry (Steinberg 1981), this small book attracted considerable criticism for saying so, particularly from academic units, but considerable support from people of all disciplines working in multidisciplinary child psychiatric teams, where inter-professional conflict was common enough to be a recurring problem. In fact there are good reasons why multidisciplinary work *should* be difficult, since if it is to represent a genuine diversity of perspectives (e.g. individually-focused *versus* family-focused treatment, or the pros and cons of medication), there is bound to be stress and strain and, in psychiatry at least, aspects of the history and development of multidisciplinary work have been undoubtedly turbulent (e.g. Parry-Jones 1986; Steinberg 1986a,b; Pichot 2000). Consultative work as pioneered and developed by Caplan provided systematic ways for different disciplines to work together on a peer basis, and we will examine whether this special characteristic could be adapted to help clinicians and patients work together as equal partners.

Are clinicians and patients 'equal', or is this a hypocritical exercise? In terms of technical knowledge and skill, doctors and patients aren't equal, and if they were there would be no point to a clinical consultation. This remains true if, for example, a doctor consults another doctor, or a psychotherapist another psychotherapist.

One person may consult another because of the other's special or wider (i.e. unequal) technical skills, while they remain equals in every other way, and it seems to me that this may apply no less to doctor (or any other clinician or therapist) and patient. As far as patient as peer is concerned, the only senses in which he or she is not a peer is if (a) illness prevents the patient being so; for example, if the patient is incapacitated or physically or mentally unwell to contribute, or if the way the patient feels leads to a request for the clinician to take charge; and (b) they do not know enough about the technicalities of the disorder or the options for treatment, despite the doctor's best efforts to make the relevant issues clear in the doctor's traditional role as teacher. These two conditions point to the great complexities in clinical care but, once again, their acknowledgement as issues, and their admissibility in thinking about how clinician and patient relate to each other, is often all that is necessary; consultation is a rational way of proceeding, not a miracle problem-solver.

Given that these obvious factors aren't in the way, the following consultative issue can be considered: *that IPC is an exercise in encouraging the other person's knowledge and skills, and raises the question of what each participant can contribute.*

Can the clinician's contribution be complemented by what the patient can do in describing the problem and deciding about treatment? Aside from the patient's role in clarifying problems and needs, patient participation in treatment itself is well established in many conditions (e.g. in digestive disorders, diabetes, asthma) and as a sine qua non in many occupational and psychological therapies. Even no more than the simple charting of symptoms can be informative for patient and clinician out of all proportion to the minimal time it takes (e.g. ticking a couple of boxes daily) and can contribute to a sense of control over the condition, for example in anxiety, obsessive–compulsive and habit disorders, as well as the possibly useful contribution of a biofeedback effect in some cases. In all these and other ways, the groundwork for self-management is there to be developed.

'Alternative' or 'complementary' therapy is a good example of an area where the patient may have wider knowledge of what is available than the mainstream practitioner. This isn't the place to attempt a review of complementary medicine, but my own experience is that, taken as a whole, it is a huge, rich mixture of good advice and bad, the cranky and the brilliant, the trivial, the commonsensical and the important. If a patient asks a clinician whether there are alternative therapies for a particular condition (or to prevent one), what kind of response is he or she likely to get? 'Alternative' therapies and all kinds of self-help and health-promotion strategies, again ranging from the sensible to the daft, are used on so huge a scale, for good and ill, that perhaps it is time for mainstream medical training to include their comprehensive coverage, so that the clinician should be able to discuss these treatments with patients knowledgeably and discriminatingly.

Whatever the health issue, there should be clarity about the difference between *information* and *decision-making*. A doctor discussing, for example, the genetic loading of an inherited disorder or the pros and cons of a particular drug treatment or surgical operation can put the known facts plus his or her own judgement of the balance of probabilities before the patient, who then makes up his or her mind. In that the patient may not be able to make his mind up easily, the doctor then moves to another aspect of the consultative mode, where the task is not yet more information-giving or opinion-giving (that having been done), but helping the patient think through how and perhaps with whom to make a decision.

IPC's role in deciding who is in the best position to do what

We have seen that consultation is not only about what patient and doctor can do, but what working with the doctor's colleagues can contribute too. With the focus on the patient, there is the new question of the contribution the patient's family and network can make. Again, this is well established in a patchy kind of way, but consultative skills can pull such things together more systematically, make them more central and in focus, and lay the foundations for information-sharing, coordination and mutual education.

What is available 'outside' can be notoriously difficult to keep up to date with – for example – who in a given locality is properly qualified, well regarded and available to provide counselling, or stress management, or an aspect of health education or home care, but it would be reasonable to expect the front-line practitioner or a colleague to have some knowledge of how to go about finding out; it is something clinician and client should be able to swap notes about. Awareness of what family members and friends could be asked (by the patient) to do is part of exploring the patient's network. Whether or not they are able or willing to help is a second question; the first is simply that the notion is on the agenda. If serial examination of this demonstrates only a patient's actual or emotional isolation, or a relative's unhelpfulness, that too is worth knowing.

All this is part of what a family practitioner will be interested in knowing about in any case; systems consultation provides the more general strategy into which this kind of knowledge fits. Thinking along these lines itself adds to the chain reaction of useful enquiry; does this patient need a lawyer rather than a counsellor? A different job rather than stress management? The housing department or some other office in the local authority? A spiritual adviser? There is a whole range of people, services and benefits that are heavily used by a minority and not known about by many. To reiterate a point made earlier, the point is not for the clinician to go through such options as if by checklist, but simply to have in the back of the mind the image of the total person functioning in his or her total environment, alongside the other image of the patient as an illustration from *Gray's Anatomy*.

IPC and the psychology of consultation

Feelings matter, because they affect judgements and decision-making as well as personal wellbeing. In the previous chapter we discussed how the emotional issues in consultation included attention to how much is, so to speak, personal and within oneself, to be resolved in one's own way; and how much is related to the work, and appropriate to a consultative approach of one kind or another. In that context I mentioned that the experience of consultation can enhance consultation with oneself, so that the clinician experienced in this way can – ideally – sift through feelings about a patient or a clinical interview and ask not 'who's to blame' (that's assuming negative feelings) but rather, 'how much of this am I contributing, and how much is the client?' In many clinical situations the clinician should at least consider himself or herself responsible for the atmosphere of a consultation. At least, a willingness to start out from that reflective, objectively self-questioning position may help highlight the fact that sometimes it *is* the client's responsibility, and then, still following the rules of consultation, the question is, first, can clinician and patient stand aside from the presenting problem and discuss whether they are able to have a positive discussion about it? And if not, whether continuing may not be workable. Ordinarily, unfortunately, the archetypal undercurrent of the patient's dependence on the doctor, and the doctor feeling in return that he or she has got to come up with the goods or otherwise deemed some kind of failure, is so powerful that standing aside to review the rules of engagement can seem impossible. But it isn't, and if patient autonomy is to be encouraged and enhanced, either side should be able to draw attention not only to the content of working together but also to the practicalities of doing so. It should not be that difficult, I think, to step aside from a 'stuck' clinical consultation (to step over to the 'other side', or 'offstage', as it were), suggest a breathing space, and ask: 'how are we doing?' If badly, that needs to be acknowledged.

What is required, as in any consultation, is to consult with the consultee about progress and to be alert to the possibility of the focus getting lost. Another test of good consultation is that role-reversal should be possible. If the clinician asks the client to pause for a moment and contribute to seeing whether they are getting anywhere useful, the *clinician* is for that moment the consultee, and the *client* the consultant. It does not matter if roles are exchanged in the interest of dealing with a particular aspect of a health matter, so long as the difference is clear, because in the clinical aspect of the task it is the clinician's authority that is paramount, and in the consultative aspect of the task it is that of the patient.

Conclusions: more consultation, less therapy

If the consultative way of getting the necessary information together and reaching decisions is the best guarantor of maximising patient autonomy, this requires as much clarity as possible about the difference between the clinical component, where it is the clinician's authority and responsibility for information-providing and opinion-giving, and the consultative component, where it is the consultee's authority and responsibility to reach a decision, bringing in his own knowledge, assumptions and approaches as he wishes. Clinical skills are for the technically trained specialist; consultative skills are for everyone.

In discussing other ways the medical consultation could operate, I cannot help wondering if we can learn something from that much-maligned profession, the law. While the traditional medical enquiry is about what the clinician can diagnose in the patient, and treat, the essence of the client–lawyer relationship, at least the place from which they start, is something like: 'given all that, what can we do? What are all the options?' I think we would have an equivalent conversation with an architect or builder if the house fell down. Could that kind of way into a problem be usefully transplanted into medical work?

The 'medical model' and consultation

I have referred several times to that convenient straw man, the 'medical model', usually used to stereotype doctors as authoritarian and paternalistic and seeing disorder and treatment only in biological terms. No doubt some are, as are some who make this assertion while quite often themselves employing the real essence of the medical model, which it seems me is less to do with specifically biological aetiology and therapy and more to do with *the process of diagnosing something wrong with the client*. I repeat this distinction here, because of the rather large number of approaches and practitioners who claim to be offering an alternative to the 'medical model' while actually employing it, albeit that their own conceptual models are psychological or psychodynamic (Tyrer and Steinberg 2005). Even self-styled holistic or humanistic practitioners can employ surprisingly narrowly focused criteria for disorder and methods for treatment.

Approaches which do not do this include client-centred counselling or psychotherapy (e.g. Rogers 1951; Silverstone 1993), and which are consultative in style, and to an extent family therapy practitioners, although what family therapy has abandoned in terms of individual diagnosis some family therapists have replaced by very definite notions of what they consider to be family pathology.

Whatever the reader may conclude about the pros and cons of systems consultation, I hope I have made the case for it being the genuine antithesis of the medical model in that it asks not what is wrong with the other person, but about what is right, and about what he or she sees as right or wrong about their situation, moreover as a joint enquiry. This attention to socio-cultural networks and immediate relationships (including the doctor–patient relationship) will often not be sufficient, which is why the consultative approach is suggested as something to supplement clinical enquiry, not as a second line of enquiry but a parallel one. As to 'patient autonomy', systems consultation would not be able to proceed coherently without it.

The role of writing it down

In Chapter 11 the narrative magic of words in therapy is discussed. The transforming power of the spoken word in any therapeutic conversation applies also to the written word (Steinberg 2004a), notably in how we write letters to and about clients. As well as being informative they can be reminders of something undertaken, agreements, or items for a future agenda; they link one consultation with the next and are tangible tokens and literal contributions to maintaining therapeutic momentum, and have a potentially important function in enhancing the status and role of the patient. Unlike conversation, which is transient and open to retrospective modification, a letter is there in black and white and can be reflected upon, commented on, discussed, reviewed, challenged, treasured, or even regretted, in the varying circumstances and moods and changes of mind to which clinician and client are entitled. In all these ways a letter, either addressed to a patient or copied to them, has many of the inherent qualities of consultation, because unlike the session to which it refers, it remains wide open, negotiable. I think we should treat letter writing as a serious skill, and part of our training (Steinberg 2000b).

CHAPTER 11

Medicine as art, art as medicine: the humanities in healthcare

- Medicine and the arts.
- Healthcare stories and the power of words.
- Reviewing the story so far.
- The humanities in healthcare: a different kind of narrative.

Medicine and the arts

One of the more surprising and encouraging developments of recent times has been the proliferation of the arts and humanities within hospitals and other medical institutions. Kaye (1997) identifies as pivotal in this development the outcome of the Carnegie Trust's inquiry, under the chairmanship of Sir Richard Attenborough (Attenborough 1985) into the role of the arts in the National Health Service and the social services. It noted the ad hoc use of the arts as optional extras, and proposed instead that they should have an integral role in healing and caring. It is important to distinguish these developments from those of art therapy, important as they are, because the latter have tended to focus on the treatment of individual disability or disorder, notably in psychiatry and learning problems, using art techniques, while the arts in healthcare movement has been more about the total healing environment, particularly in general medical care.

Before 1985 and especially since, there have been many accounts of the importance of the arts in promoting an environment conducive to recovery (e.g. Revans 1962; Ulrich 1984, 1992; Langer 1989; Miles 1994; Wilkinson 2000; review by Staricoff and Loppert 2003). On the one hand there is an accumulating impression and increasing evidence that patients' morale is improved, benefiting their health and recovery, that staff morale improves too, with tangible benefits for staff recruitment and retention, that neglect and vandalism is discouraged, and that, in Kaye's words, there is a 're-calibration of the relationship between patient, staff and environment' (Kaye 1997). On the other hand, there is also the view that in all settings a pleasing environment is good in itself, enhances a sense of life being worthwhile and that one is being cared for, and why should we spend many millions on factory-like, indeed barracks-like, clinics when we could spend much the same making them beautiful? In this context art galleries, museums, libraries and theatres, whatever their content, tend to be carefully designed, decorated and well maintained, while many areas of many hospitals are ill-decorated, scruffy and sometimes filthy (*see* page 167). Does art, whether 'good' or 'bad', raise our sights?

The case can be made that art is good for you; certainly there is evidence that feeling good can have a direct impact on the neuroimmune systems and the healing process (e.g. Ornstein and Sobel 1988), and even if we can not yet handle such suppositions with clinical precision they seem worth pursuing. Elsewhere (Steinberg 2004a, and forthcoming) I have argued that the components of the artistic impulse and appreciation are literally vitally necessary, in our evolution, in our personal development and in normal, sane functioning. To say that art is 'good for you' is not the same as saying we all need art therapy; rather, I would suggest that the relationship between art therapy and art in the environment is equivalent to, say, that between physiotherapy and physical activity.

Art is something we are all qualified to comment on, wherever we find it; we may enjoy or dislike it, be impressed by it or baffled by it, staff and patients alike; it can provide a common, accessible atmosphere. This may seem a smallish point until you compare it with the power of architecture and design to communicate: it may be to impress; to give the appearance of ancient strength and authority (lots of columns and steps) or forward-looking modernity; to convey importance, power and prestige; even to intimidate. Organisational systems can present a kind of importance, the separateness of its personnel, its distractedness from your problem to higher things; obviously in its uniforms and signwriting, in its 'corporate image' and slogans, but also in its chaos and busy-ness, its attention focused on crisis management and the telephone: too busy to see you, too busy to talk, too busy in fact to treat you.

The arts, compared with high-tech science, are still in comparison relatively innocent in such respects, less easily controlled, more unpredictable, more demotic. And priesthoods, especially our latter-day high-tech priesthoods, can be as uneasy about the demotic as the demonic. Perhaps the arts can bring us all down to earth, healthcare personnel and patients alike, stop us in our tracks, invite us to think what we are doing here, in this hospital or that clinic.

I like Kaye's words, quoted above; that the arts may recalibrate the relationship between staff, patients and environment. The arts might also contribute to raising and widening the level of the debate from survival to something worth doing well together. I think this bears a relationship to systems consultation, which is also about standing back and taking another, wider and different look, one that allows for going with the innovatory as well as falling back on the conventional. In relation to what we make of the arts, from poetry to pop lyrics, from cartoons to 'gallery art' we are all experts; I think the phrase 'I know what I like' is an honourable one, albeit treated sniffily by art's priesthood. And if we go a little deeper into what it takes to appreciate or make art, this generates the kind of receptive, open, imaginative and creative frame of mind that may help the health enterprise too. The balance between control and spontaneity the artist in any field must achieve in relation to his or her work seems to operate around a very different fulcrum from the control of the scientist and the technologist, and may teach us something valuable and enduring beyond the undoubted utility of this year's 'hard facts'.

The history: the function of narrative and the power of words

On the one hand it may not seem obvious why the notion of narrative – story-telling – should be introduced here, and yet the taking of the patient's history is one of the cornerstones of clinical care. The patient brings his or her story to the clinical consultation, and the clinician, from a knowledge of many other stories (such as what happens with cancer or cardiac disease) listens, and adds to the story, including the alternative endings, depending on stories about different kinds of clinical intervention: more stories. We see these stories in the basements of old medical libraries: shelves of tattered textbooks and rows of leather-bound and long-forgotten papers, surveys and reports, which served their function well at the time, tend to wear out; but it does seem that other kinds of stories, for example about the philosophy of science, or biographical and fictional work by therapists and scientists and patients, seem to be what keeps the subject alive and capable of taking on new information. It is, in a way, the 'other', more earthy and fertile, side of the medical literature.

Elsewhere I have described the work of the psychotherapist as like being a kind of editor, suggesting that the unhappy client's history, in effect his autobiography, his whole notion of himself, may benefit from some rethinking and revision, some additions, deletions and reworking (Steinberg 2000b, 2004a). Kleinman (1988) has described how illness and the experience of illness is shaped by our social and cultural environment, that there are 'illness narratives' (having a cold; having a heart attack; going mad), while Higgs (2003) reminds us, from his experience of the pioneering Balint groups in general practice, that the doctor's tale contributes to the culture-bound, environmental and also to the psychological understanding of illness (Higgs, 2003; Balint 1968). Frank, in an account entitled *The Wounded Storyteller* (1997), has described how in modern Western culture the personal experience of being ill is overwhelmed by the highly technical, complex organisation of diagnosis and treatment, in which specialists using a special language reinterpret their distress and pain in their own terms. Frank says, 'illness becomes the circulation of stories, professionals and lay, but not all stories are equal'. We have a dilemma here for clinical science, in that the specialist's story may be better: for example, I think that some of my (and my colleagues') stories about schizophrenia or depression are 'better' than the stories of some of my patients about schizophrenic and depressive experiences. Similarly, given a mysterious pain I may well prefer the surgeon's and radiologists's stories (the latter nicely illustrated) to my own. But for a whole host of reasons, to do with diagnosis, treatment and the process of healing, the patient's story is *also* important (the clinician as co-author, not just editor) and this is where attention to the other side of medical care, with its other language, comes in.

Launer (2002), in his account of primary medical care based on narrative methods, distinguishes between the *knowledge-based stance* of the doctor as expert and the *narrative-based stance* which can be shared by doctor and patient and which challenges technical expertise without being allowed to undermine it: in other words, acknowledging the value of both (Launer 1996, 2002). Higgs and others discuss not only the use of narrative in therapy, but the importance of the arts in widening our capacity for describing things from without and within, objectively and intuitively (Higgs 2003; Kirklin and Richardson 2003). Perhaps the arts can play their part in promoting health and preventing illness in a way complementary to being normally physically active, with an association between good health and being creative, innovative, positive, imaginative, optimistic and open to stimulus being worth hypothesising and worth research.

Words and narrative have power. If anything in the down-to-earth and natural things we are discussing deserves the epithet 'magic', it is surely the power of words (Steinberg 2000b, 2004a). The very word 'grammar' derives from *grammaire*, Old French for a book of magic spells. For the magic to work you have to get the spelling and the narrative right, rather like getting the prescription right. We still use a magic symbol on our prescriptions – the Rx sign, representing a prayer to Jove that the medicine may help more than harm, and protecting the patient; in these modern days it is printed lest the prescriber forgets to write it. The power of words is partly because we naturally take them for granted (though as we have seen, psychoanalysts and deconstructionists don't), and through the culture they shape *us* as much as we shape them, something that is consistent with much recent study of the development of language (e.g. Dennett 1991, Pinker 1994, 2002). Words, spoken or written, indeed any sort of notation, share this potency. Words carry more than meets the eye, or ear: they are like packets of communication, containing multiple meanings, ambiguities and implications, and when therapist and client exchange even ordinary words, emotional resonances accompany them.

Poesis means making: creating. The message, I think, of the use of narrative in healthcare is cautionary as well as creative: the methods of science have given us half the story. We, whether as clinician or as patient, need to provide the other half, and we have to be as good storytellers and poets as are the tellers of scientific tales to get the narrative right.

In this way Launer's, Franks' and others' notions of narrative in therapeutic work take us some of the way towards an understanding of systems consultation, though not the whole way. The therapeutic-type account, the kind of biographical and poetic narrative I have described as benefiting from editing and joint authorship, helps make something of both the clinician's and the patient's position and self-perceptions. However, a new or renewed mode of story-telling is needed to make sense of the systems in the environment in which clinician and patient operate, and its characteristics owe more to the literature of exploration, travel writing and even, perhaps, the best of investigative journalism. I think the joint enquiry of systems consultation is like this.

The story so far: the system consultant's tale

1   To take up the threads of the story as we left it in Chapter 10: healthcare, its practitioners and its consumers constitute a vast and growing industry. In outlook, ambition and achievements it may be asked whether its wonders ever cease. What is needed is a whole new philosophy of medicine and care.

2   Healthcare's basic premise is the concept that something in the human body and mind has gone wrong in its anatomy or functioning, and that if this is sufficiently and properly researched techniques can be developed to put it right; and more than this, prevent it from happening in the first case. It is a bold prospectus, justified by results again and again but always generating new problems. International and government agencies have already begun speculating about the state of perfect health.

3   As it isn't universally taken for granted that all this is a good thing, it needs to be said that modern healthcare science and practice have been enormously successful within the terms of their own general prospectus (point 2 above) and deserve the status, role and the resources devoted

to them. Systems consultation however reveals the nine-tenths of the iceberg that remains underneath.

4   Medicine's very success has sucked into its slipstream a whole new world of need of every shape and kind, until huge areas of human distress and social and personal mismanagement and bad fortune are increasingly classed as disorders, and the number and type of therapists of every description grow. Healthcare's cultural status is such that it is not now thought mad to patch up gaps in services with counselling. (Where the police have led will the post office, railways and fire brigade follow? Might we soon have couselling about the non-availability of healthcare?)

5   There are many accounts of the extent to which we live in an increasingly 'therapised' culture (e.g. Fitzpatrick 2000; Furedi 2004; but see also Samuel Butler's novel *Erewhon* (1922)). It seems largely a product of high technology and prosperity, and perhaps the failure of traditional cultural values, but impoverished cultures seem to aspire to our model too. We do seem engaged as much in patient making as in patient treating.

6   The advance of medical science is fine, but like any healthy development needs to be balanced by counter-argument. For reasons given in the last chapter we cannot trust the 'anti-medical model' movements to take charge of the brakes because to a large extent it seems that they are irredeemably part of the diagnose-and-treat industry themselves; and good luck to them, but I would suggest that their claim to be notably alternative, humanistic and patient-centred and to 'really' speak on the patient's behalf be tested against the principles of the peer–peer oriented, consultative approach.

7   Systems consultation is neither pro- nor anti- the 'medical model', indeed is inherently open to paying attention to the positions of all of its passing collaborators, allies and competitors including their philosophies and values (for an account of which, *see* Pattison and Pill 2004). In a sense it is a-moral (which is not the same as immoral), though as we have seen, the consultant has no obligation to help with something he or she considers unethical, counterproductive or mad. The proposition in this book is not that the clinical approach is flawed, but that it is incomplete. Linking clinical and systems components of consultation as a dual approach provides an effective way of making the most of specialist skills on the one hand and what the client wants and can do on the other; and both sides learn from the encounter.

8   None of this is entirely new. Many clinicians (and other experts) are good *because* they use a consultative kind of style. Good lawyers, accountants, designers, craftsmen and psychotherapists do. The point, however, is that it could help negotiation in, and about, the rapidly advancing medical world of today and the near future if consultation skills were more widely understood and applied.

Talking the same language: how the arts and humanities can help

It is clearly in everyone's interests, in healthcare, for representatives of all the many different disciplines involved to be capable of working together. The practical value of inter-professional and organisational consultation practice, the rationale for its development, is *because* true multidisciplinary work (as opposed to its pretence, or lip-service to it) is not easy.

Talking the same language as our clientele is potentially difficult too. As I mentioned earlier (page 79), the illusion of mutual understanding can be even more profound when people believe they are formally communicating in the same language; than when circumstances necessitate the help of translators.

I will outline a few of the ways in which learning from the arts can help our work in healthcare.

The power of the clown in our culture

In his description of the use of narrative in primary care, Launer (2002) referred to its role as that of the court jester, whose traditional role was to challenge authority with wit and yet without sabotaging it. This reminds me of Leach's witty but sobering idea of how cultures cope with innovators – by consigning them to prisons, mental hospitals or universities. To this I would add – to the arts. (A really peculiar and unsafe-seeming occurrence in one's local high street would probably make one think of these three or four means of explanation, if not disposal.) The artist occupies an ambiguous role in society – both as the magical genius, an iconic and even godlike figure, and as the useless fool. The alternative archetypes are the 'star' on the one hand, advancing up the red carpet, and the outsider, the pavement artist, on the other. Art might achieve anything, and nothing. Science, on the other hand, proceeds slowly, solidly and with caution, conducted by people trained as scientists, and its achievements are slow and hard-won; scientific 'truth' is discarded for other truths in a decade, in a generation or in a hundred years. Aesthetic truths may last a week, if they don't misfire and burn out in the course of one performance, or become eternal. The one is focused, objective, measurable, the product of convergent thinking and measurement. The other is open to anything, intuitive, impressionistic, the product of divergent thinking. We know we need the former, but we also need the latter, not only for the wider picture, but because we know that while intuition, like nature, is wasteful, it also provides the raw material for innovation. Innovation is needed, of course, not only in research and development but also for the unique qualities of the individual person's case. Ideas, observation and measurement may operate in a circular system, but discovery is often initiated by intuition and a first idea which *then* leads to the findings which confirm or refute it.

In this sense everyone is some kind of artist, and we need to cultivate the artist's perception and attitude to make sense of the other side of medical care, whether it is in terms of insight or understanding each other, or the crazy environments and institutions we build for ourselves. We need the jester, not to mock destructively, but to help us be a little sceptical about the nature of illusion; the jester's traditional power was less in what he said than in how he looked: all dressed up, like the King and Court.

Contributions from psychodynamic theory, mythology and anthropology

Psychoanalytic theory (the Freudian precursor of psychodynamic theory in general) is vast, and the thread I want to draw out of it in this context is small. Its detractors have called it no more than a mythology, and Freud more a literary figure than a scientist, as if these assertions spoil his story. Curiously, the detractors of mythology sometimes seem to speak as if myths had a kind of historical reality in biblical times or in ancient Greece or Rome, and are now out of date. But myths are the products of real, live brains and minds, stories men and women conjured up from their imaginations to make sense of their worlds and as cautionary tales. They are psychological as well as historical or 'classical' phenomena, and they have evolutionary significance (e.g. Stevens 1982). In individual lives they have developmental significance, and all kinds of narrative, including the particularly potent psychoanalytical narrative, can throw light on the emotional side of what goes on within ourselves and between us and our colleagues and clients. Freud's work focused on the unconscious influence of biologically primitive and emotionally immature impulses on conscious motivation and behaviour, and this is as universal as the weather, even in the most scientifically and rationally based health clinics and departments, among staff as well as patients. Brown's (1961) and Wollheim's (1971) accounts are short and clear, and Tyrer and Steinberg (2005) provide an outline summary. The literary figure Harold Bloom captures the reciprocity of science, myth and art when he comments in his critical account of Freud that 'throwing Freud out will not get rid of him, because he is inside us. His mythology of the mind has survived his supposed science and his metaphors are impossible to evade.' (Bloom 2002) In that tantalising and complex reciprocity between human development and human culture, the Freudian narrative arises from the biological roots of our minds and returns to contribute to our mental processes and our relationships. It is a narrative – among many others – that is told and heard again and again in the clinic.

The paediatrician and psychoanalyst DW Winnicott described art as having many of the qualities of what psychoanalysts know as transitional objects, namely a thing, person or relationship which holds a situation while powerful conflicting feelings concerning it are resolved one way or another (*see* page 47). Winnicott was describing parent–infant relationships, and while the similarities between this and aspects of the therapeutic and the consultative setting could be argued, it is also possible to see the arts, including particularly narrative and drama, as also managing to be at the same time both containing and exploratory, and capable of holding the ambiguity of a situation (e.g. not knowing what to think, what to do or whom to trust) with the possibility of an ultimate resolution (*see* Winnicott 1965, 1988). This psychological model is consistent with aspects of art therapy. Might it also contain the seeds of an explanatory model for the arts providing nurturing and healing environments in healthcare?

For other contributions to the art, science, mythology and anthropology of how we relate to each other, in sickness and in health, I would recommend the writings of Jung (*see* pages 36 *et seq*, and Jung 1964; Stevens 1990; Campbell 1974); and to relate these to healthcare's history, I would recommend the writings on shamanism, for example Vitebsky's (1995) introduction.

Attachment theory and creativity

Attachment theory was described earlier (pages 45 *et seq*). Based on psychodynamic theory and observations of the behaviour of human and animal families, it generated a model very like Winnicott's, showing how, in a relationship, a safe base from which to explore could be generated. Both the 'safe base' and the 'exploration' referred to real exploration in real and potentially dangerous territory, but this also provides a powerful metaphorical model for exploring ideas and feelings. There are few so alarmed or enraged as those whose fundamental ideas and attitudes are seriously challenged, because the survival of the self and its integrity, indeed sanity, may feel threatened. Handling this, if only enough to comprehend (rather than dismiss) what the other person is getting at, is increasingly problematic in highly specialised, highly politicised cultures like our own. It requires tolerance of such ambiguous circumstances as (for example) empathising with the other person's views without having to agree with them, presumably because we have enough confidence in our own narrative without fearing that it will be compromised by taking another person's tale seriously. I mention it here because I think it describes a therapeutic skill and the kind of strength it takes to be a competent consultant or consultee; because it is an art, and like art capable of being creative in the face of danger; and because it seems to me that the themes of attachment theory throw light on it.

Investigating, discovering, and writing a different story: the power of serial questions

The traditional medical narrative is a familiar one from our teachers and our textbooks: take for example the symptoms and signs of an illness, like, say, meningitis, appendicitis or snakebite; nothing is clearer, culturally, ethically, professionally and legally, than the doctor confirming the diagnosis and prescribing what's needed.

However, much of modern medicine is less and less like this. A smaller proportion of the whole is now clear-cut, or capable of swift resolution with acute medical or surgical care. Even an overdose, so romanticised in novels and at least the older films, can also now become a clinical and ethical mess involving emergency rooms (sometimes with punch-ups), 'disposal' problems between the ER and half a dozen wards in hospital and the local psychiatric hospital, the police, social services and the patient's family and friends, all as potential contributors to the crisis as well as potential sources of help. The sick child, again a potent traditional symbol for many entering the caring professions, may now present as the truculent son of a truculent and divided family arguing with the clinician the pros and cons of medication, while the clinician has much the same arguments with her colleagues and within herself.

The clinical consultation – establishing an overdose of antidepressants, or attention-deficit hyperactivity disorder – provides an incomplete narrative; the story has to be continued with a systems dialogue, enquiring into who else should be doing what, and whether they can be helped to even see it, let alone do it. The kinds of serial question asked may lead into all sorts of unexpected territory. Beginning with a disturbed child in a children's home, we have seen that the answer may be that the staff could cope if a manager helped them with their rotas, their training and supervision, even with their pay and conditions. We have even seen how people don't always have the room and the time in which to do their jobs. People who may even be as yet uninvolved may need to be contacted, told the story, asked if they agree with the newly emerging narrative, asked to take a role, asked to see it through.

I hope it is clear what this all has to do with narrative, and the arts. The kinds of situation that arise in healthcare are so complex, kaleidoscopic and chaotic that more than one story can be used as an explanation or description of what is happening. In fact, many more. All sorts of things can determine the preferred narrative – the one that gets published, so to speak – and many of them, even the alleged 'scientific' accounts, and certainly the organisational ones, are often largely arbitrary, and entail substantial editing and selection. In systems consultation, consultant and consultee explore alternative descriptions and explanations – a different story. Looking more widely for additional and different kinds of evidence and writing a new account as joint authors, is legitimate, time-honoured and respectable in both science and the arts. But it may be that in healthcare not all of our present policy-makers, administrators and scientists are up to it. It may be that for the kind of courage, experimentation, imagination, innovation, optimism, generosity, eccentricity, intuition and audacity, and for the capacity for thinking the unthinkable that is going to be needed, we will also have to look to the example of the arts.

CHAPTER 12

Systems consultation and the other side of common sense

- A short summary: the consultative attitude.
- Common *vs* uncommon sense.
- Simplicity *vs* complexity.
- Good intentions about the 'good doctor'.
- Consultative approaches and healthcare policies.
- Minding the gaps.

A short summary

If you've started the book here, that's all right; the theme throughout is the advantage of circular systems approaches over linear.

Systems consultation involves discussing with the client, or consultee, his position, predicament, ideas, wishes, information, skills and the other resources available in his relationships and his situation, all in relation to a perceived problem or issue. This is often about problem solving, but the 'problem' can also be how to improve or develop something – health, of course, but perhaps training, or work with colleagues. As consultant you may be working with a group – your consultee's colleagues; or your own colleagues.

All this casts a very wide net in relation to the external social and cultural systems of which the consultee and yourself are part. It is the obverse and partner of *clinical consultation*, which is about the no less complicated system within the patient, from facts and metaphors about how the mind works to his neural pathways, his circulatory, respiratory, digestive and metabolic systems, immune and reproductive systems and his blood, bones, joints, muscles and his skin.

I am aware of the paradoxical problem, here, of contrasting clinical consultation with systems consultation in order to then bring them both together. The point is they are both forms of systems consultation, one, as said, paying attention to the systems within, including individual psychic systems, and the other to external systems, including the psychology of relationships and institutions. The account by Pendleton and others about new developments in the clinical consultation (Pendleton *et al.* 2003) is an important step in this kind of direction, but while it provides an enlightened approach to work with patients, it doesn't encompass the extent of the social and psychological networks described here.

Bearing in mind Wall's first rate advice to handle language with care (Wall 2003), and having moved from the terminology of 'inter-professional consultation' to 'consultation for everybody', and emphasised the difference between the one and the other, one may still hope that when the latter has matured as much as the former, and after an appropriately lengthy engagement, they might undergo some kind of meiosis and reproduction together, and bud off something good and new.

It's all very complicated, these two systems, especially when we face the fact of the constantly changing dynamic interaction between the two, and between the systems they engage with; but we would not expect life and the politics of life to be simple.

Systems consultation and clinical consultation, taken together, provide neither easy answers nor overarching theories but a pragmatic way into all this complexity, and one that takes your consultee or client with you, as a necessary partner. They are experts too; few exploring strange territory would turn down the services of a willing local guide.

When, where and how

Giving an account of the intricacies and twists and turns that happen in pursuing consultative approaches makes it seem that systems consultation, or systems and clinical consultation together, means having very extended and sometimes repeated conversations, with rooms to be booked and dates and times to be fixed. It can, but it has not been the primary purpose of this book to encourage every senior healthcare worker to make time and space for regular consultative work. Rather, my hope is that by giving an account of how consultative approaches can be pursued systematically, and with pukka, formal consultative sessions becoming both the ideal model and the occasional experience of practitioners (perhaps for particular problems or issues, or in training), that the consultative approach might be seen as a kind of style, or voluntary mindset; a system-side manner to go alongside the bedside manner.

'Being consultative' could then be slipped into as if it were a change of conversational gear, whether acknowledged in a few phrases, or in a few minutes spent during a primarily clinical conversation to look at the matter from another perspective. This could be extended, between consenting adults of course, into a more focused meeting if that seemed useful. What matters, I think, is the style of a consultative dialogue, its few but quite important rules, the curiosity and empathy it requires, and its acknowledgement of the wider, multidimensional and dynamic matrix in which doctor, patient and the art, science and organisation of healthcare are embedded.

Consultation, and common and uncommon sense

By one of those curious coincidences that might possibly qualify as a Jungian synchronicity, I am writing this note about common sense in the study of the house that was Lord Lister's home 150 years ago. The day's news is dominated by more government initiatives on methicillin-resistant staphylococcus aureus (MRSA), the 'superbug' killing and disabling thousands of people currently catching the infection in dirty hospitals. When Joseph Lister tried to persuade doctors to wash their hands and remove or cover up their dirty street clothes when in the operating theatre he was regarded as a crank. The common sense of the time was that pus-stained, bloodied clothing was the mark of the busy and therefore experienced surgeon. Micro-organisms weren't quite discovered, but Lister suspected something toxic and damaging was literally in the air when wounds became infected and patients died of septicaemia, rather as astroscientists have drawn inferences from clues and predicted new planets before they have been found. Against doubts and resistance, the new common sense came in: henceforth – from around Victorian times – the hallmark of the hospital became the smell of disinfectant, starched linen and polished floors, with a fierce Matron or Ward Sister on the look-out for dust and dirt, indeed untidiness generally.

Dirt has been defined as matter in the wrong place. Thus even untidiness – a coat on a bed – in one of those old-fashioned wards would have been suspect, whether or not a connection could be proved with infection. Tidiness; cleanliness being next to Godliness; freshly laundered uniforms; polished floors; washing your hands; order; authority; it kind of went together, and while 'germs' were by then part of common sense, the rest of this package gradually became associated with old-fashioned arbitrary authority, and washing your hands somewhat passé. Out it went, along with strictly supervised cleanliness and tidiness. Enter MRSA, no slave to fashion, and where methicillin failed a paper war began, with statements, posters, plans, initiatives, programmes, projects, Infection Czars, plus bottles of alcogel on nurses' belts and around doctors' necks, since staff were too busy to wash their hands at the widely dispersed wash-hand basins, and then the whole hand-drying business had become complicated by towels being dirty, air-dryers slow and boring, and everything contracted-out anyway. The new common sense does not include anything about Lister or the history of medicine, but is more an attempt to connect control of infection with command and control generally, the new magic, because while we can no longer trust such authority figures as Matrons and Ward Sisters, administrators instructed by politicians instructed in turn by committees expect to command our respect. Had Joseph Lister himself attempted to consult someone about it, and noted the important rule about going in at the right level, the discovery that *no-one* was in charge of the ward (although there were innumerable bosses) would have told him all he needed to know. Instead, different kinds of needs of different hierarchies are met by a high rate of turnover of staff, superspecialisation (communications nurse, liaison nurse, IT information nurse), visitors coming and going and sitting on beds in their ordinary clothes, and patients being whizzed from specialist ward to specialist ward (to get the 'best possible' care) all meant that under the new common sense *no-one* was in charge; indeed no one could possibly be wise enough to supervise all those experts. One consultant, recently, was able to insist on such measures as having clothes pegs for street clothes outside the ward, and fresh white coats inside, patients staying in one place instead of forever being buzzed around, no sitting on beds, etc., and as a result dramatically reduced MRSA infection in 'his' ward, and made it into the newspapers. Thus we advance, in slowly turning cycles. Here's something to research: might a really good theatrical production or other display about Joseph Lister's work, organised by a hospital's arts department, and inserted into the training programmes of all staff, have impact on dealing with MRSA?

Common sense is that which most people take for granted – it is *the* common sense of how things are and should be done, and in the complex modern world a generally held common sense is probably gone forever. Certainly, a theatrical production as part of science teaching is not common sense.

What is correct is now the final common path of what the political leadership of the day, the science of the moment and today's media tell us or sell us, and to a large extent it is a contradictory and phenomenally costly muddle held together by hype and illusion. There is no longer the possibility of a reliable authoritative source, and even mistakes are fudged over and made subject to a new narrative and a rewritten history.

What makes sense over any given issue may now need to be whatever can be renegotiated at ground level, and in healthcare, systems consultation allied to traditional clinical work may be the way to do it. It would seem to be a small-scale development, but one capable – if effective – of replication; and having no limit to the kinds of question it could put about the whole health and care complex, there would be no obvious limit to what it could reveal.

Simplicity to complexity and back again

In these pages there has been an ambiguity about complexity and simplicity. On the one hand I have presented systems consultation as starting out from relatively simple sets of questions, such as 'Who is concerned about what?' 'Who has the necessary information?' 'Who is in a position to help?' and the key mantra 'What is wanted, what is needed and what is possible?', with consultant and consultee pursuing such basic, even naive, questions serially and with persistence.

On the other hand, it is clear that the answers to such questions lead down pathways of labyrinthine complexity and which don't respect institutionalised boundaries. From the systems perspective, problem clarifying and problem solving is the issue, not territory. As we have seen, we may start out from problems in managing diabetes mellitus and find not a metabolic problem or a pharmacological issue but a problem in motivation or family psychodynamics; a 'seriously disturbed child' jumps the diagnostic tracks and becomes instead an issue of poor or overstretched administration or a problem in recruitment, training or the rostering of care staff; an 'intractable case' turns out to be a mixture of dispute and misunderstanding between health workers, or sometimes individual ignorance or bad practice, and then you may be immersed not in complex pathology but questions of confidentiality, professional relationships and ethics; a tricky case of drug dependence is reframed into a problem with a counsellor's job description and the design of her office.

But on the third hand, I suggest that if we, as clinicians and therapists, dare to face the whole multi-factorial, dynamic, chaotic range that constitutes the inevitable complexities of healthcare, we will eventually come up with simpler solutions, albeit that the answers may come up in someone else's field. But it depends on what we call 'simple'; one person's apparently simple solution can be another person's complex nightmare. At a clinical level we may prescribe simple solutions and go home reasonably content with the day's work, while as said earlier our patients take home a doggy bag of leftovers, unanswered and unasked questions. Systems consultation tracks back through the mess and the complexity to look for *anything* that could be better understood or usefully be changed. But getting there can be complicated, because pursuing consultative questions leads us off the beaten track – away from the usual channels – and into territory and across boundaries that we are often encouraged to avoid.

The people we work with

The problems patients present aren't the only things that deserve attention. Working with our colleagues can generate problems too. Earlier I suggested that the Tower of Babel was a myth whose relevance continues to the present in institutions, services and teams, where people with very different training, motivation, temperament and who use different conceptual models of the healthcare job have to work together while speaking quite different languages. To refer back also to Klein (page 45), who provided a psychodynamic model for showing why classifying things into 'totally good' or 'totally bad' may be immature or at least premature, the fact that multidisciplinary work and cross-disciplinary work is difficult, and can border on the impossible, is the price we pay for trying to comprehend very different perspectives about complex living systems. In this context I would like to think we could celebrate other people's odd temperaments and individuality as much as their professional contributions; but it isn't necessarily easy. Just as the remedy for the Kleinian split into 'good' and 'bad' is to be found in the question 'How good, and how bad?', the consultative approach provides a part solution in its interest in how much A can contribute, and how much B; and even if the answer is sometimes zero, the attitude behind the question makes it worth asking.

If that is common sense, then the kind of staff or team group described on page 85 *et seq* might be common sense too, one that focuses on helping people to work and make decisions together, the actual machinery of the working professional team. However, it is a very long way from being common sense at present.

Good intentions about the 'good doctor'

Technical competence and up-to-date knowledge (including where to find it), plus proper ethical and professional standards must be taken for granted as expectations if qualification and registration are to mean anything. Beyond this, people (including other doctors) tend to talk about 'good doctoring' in such terms as 'something unquantifiable', 'individualistic', and with 'no set formula that can be easily copied'; about 'humility', and about 'a desire to understand (the patient) in his or her entirety, rather than just grapple with symptoms' (Pemberton 2004).

A very new medical school includes the following as anticipated qualities of the effective medical graduate of the twenty-first century: to communicate well, including listening; to show empathy and be non-judgemental and reflective; to work well in teams; to have the ability to make decisions under pressure; to be able to deal with stress appropriately; to have problem-solving skills; to know their limitations and their strengths and weaknesses; to approach clinical problems holistically, appreciating personal and social dimensions as well as the biomedical basis of disease; and to develop the ability to learn from the problems experienced as the basis of a lifetime of learning (Peninsula Medical School 2005).

It is a worthy set of aims for any centre of healthcare training to aspire to, and doubtless many have similar criteria. However, while such qualities in the ideal doctor, or nurse, or therapist are taken for granted as desirable by any training authority, it is not obvious how these skills and characteristics are going to be taught. They involve feelings and attitudes, and take time to develop, and this requires some continuity of relationships with teachers and colleagues on the one hand and fellow-trainees and patients on the other. This does not easily fit in with the growing amount of specialty teaching, and the understandable importance given to knowing lots of facts. The ingredients are being poured in, as it were, many of them very fine indeed; but how will the recipients be taught how to cook?

There is no avoiding the conflict between the limited time available in medical training, and the unlimited amount there is to know. It is taken for granted that the doctor of the future needs to be prepared for a professional lifetime of keeping up to date. However, to acquire maturity as a professional the student needs also to be taught *how to continue learning from patients and from other healthcare workers about how to be a doctor*, and taken as a whole, culturally and occupationally, the working situation as it is likely to be for the forseeable future is not going to be very conducive to this. Knowing how to use systems consultation alongside clinical consultation may be one way of acquiring this sort of learning in complex, fast-changing and unstable situations.

Taking a wider view of new directions in healthcare, Plsek and his colleagues have pointed out how the greatest need for twenty-first century healthcare, which will increasingly be characterised by unpredictability and paradox, is likely to be the use of complex adaptive systems; while the greatest barrier will be the prevailing 'command and control' style of management. They propose that 'conceptual frameworks that incorporate a dynamic, emergent, creative and intuitive view of the world' must replace the traditional 'reduce and resolve' approaches to clinical care and service organisation, that care should be based on a continuing caring relationship rather than an interrupted, changing one, that transparency rather than secrecy must be paramount, that the patient should be the source of control, and that cooperation among clinicians must be a priority (e.g. Plsek and Greenhalgh 2001; Plsek and Wilson 2001).

Consultative approaches and healthcare policy

The problem with this is not so much that many presently responsible for the making and application of healthcare policies would disagree with such recommendations. Rather, they might only too readily agree, while not knowing, nor wishing to know, nor knowing how to comprehend, the full length, breadth and depth of what is being implied in terms of teaching, learning and practice. It is quite possible that the common sense of many of our current policymakers and their advisers would in fact operate *against* working along the kinds of lines Plsek and his colleagues drew up. Certainly taking an intuitive view of the world would come across to many as counterintuitive.

I am not convinced that anything big management can offer could conceivably be as effective as consultation – combined clinical and systems consultation – in (a) finding out and (b) understanding empathically what is wanted, needed and possible in healthcare. It is not the personnel involved, nor their good intentions, that is the problem; it is their perspective. Big, central management may well be best at procurement: providing buildings, advertising for staff, ordering everything from medical equipment and medication to 'hotel' supplies; but I believe a radically different relationship is needed between this kind and level of administrative work, and the determination of what kinds of building, staff and equipment are needed, and how to use them, and this would better come from a local, focused, consultative relationship between clinicians and their clientele, rather than from anywhere else.

Aside from its introduction in undergraduate and postgraduate healthcare training, how and where else might inter-professional consultative training be introduced? Its introduction, if only as an experiment, in management might be worthwhile. Occasions when an administrator seems to fully comprehend the detailed role and functioning and needs of a clinician (or the worker in any other specialised area for that matter) and vice versa, seem the exception rather than the rule. Which, when you think of it, is mad.

Other 'sites' where systems consultation would be a useful skill would be at any nodal point in the healthcare network where different services meet, new things have to be taught and learned, and dilemmas somehow resolved, and one thinks of general practitioners, as one example in healthcare, psychiatrists as another, and probably community physicians and paediatricians, and in the wider field of childcare guardians *ad litem*, those key people whose role seems more important today than ever. With social work, something seems to have come adrift, to do I think with massive overload in practice and in expectations, and the frequent concomitant of inadequate training and supervision; though if any profession would benefit its clients and itself by making systems consultation a central skill, it seems to me it would be the field of social work. Also, teachers of professionals – *any* teacher whose subject, or whose students, are multidisciplinary. How patients could learn it, or about it, to be prepared to use it as 'good consultees', for example, other than from healthcare practitioners, I am not sure; but there is such a thing as public education about health matters. Meanwhile, we have seen that consultation initiated by the practitioner has its educational component too.

Minding the gaps

The special strength and role of systems consultation is *in between*, in the gaps between the arbitrary, institutionalised distribution of specialties, special perspectives and special interests. These are in one place, while the realities of the healthcare needs of patients, and the professional needs of those who try to help, seem often to be in the spaces in between. Earlier, and somewhat reluctantly, I put the postmodern notion of deconstruction alongside psychodynamic theory as two ways of finding out what is going on whether in a clinical, training or organisational context, and – to repeat the phrase – what is wanted, needed and possible. That's where the gaps are, in lack of attention to the triad of wants, needs and possibilities in that 'other' side of medicine, and the gaps persist because we do not apply to these less straightforward aspects of healthcare the rigour associated with the best clinical inquiry.

The traditional clinical model, good as it is, just doesn't fit the new expectations of healthcare. The fact that doctors and their colleagues are expected to take on these expanding and fuzzier areas is a compliment. However, we cannot expect to simply draw a clear line between what is or is not 'medical', least of all on an arbitrary or personal basis or founded in a single preferred ideological position. This isn't just for ethical or political reasons but for reasons of practicality and logic: it simply *isn't* that clear what is or is not a disease, or an appropriate response or therapy, or the doctor's business, still less is it obvious which should be a 'correct' ethical, political or economic view. I hope at least some of the examples have demonstrated this, and that this book has shown that the consultative approach described, alongside clinical skills and just as assiduously applied, could provide a way of managing such components of healthcare's burgeoning complexity.

Precisely what it will take is for other books and other authors. It will certainly take a paradigm shift in training and healthcare strategy – but then both training and care in any case need to be robustly adaptable to whatever comes our way: hence the importance of a general system as back-up to a focused, clinical system.

It is likely to need a systematic withdrawal from the idea that big is best. Smaller, autonomous clinical and therapeutic teams and working groups could stay close to their communities, their clientele and each other, with more continuity, improving knowledge of how each other work and becoming experienced at collaborating with each other – and of course I am referring also to collaboration with non-healthcare sources of help, and with clients and potential clients. Such smaller scale enterprises would fit most of what comes medicine's way, and there is no reason why they couldn't take advantage of information technology to consult worldwide if necessary, and make the most of shared material resources too. But trying to distil *care* into vast computerised systems is hopeless.

We need to question why people in healthcare systems are perpetually on the move, whether in training, treating or being treated. The disadvantages should be weighed thoughtfully against the advantages, instead of going through on the nod to meet the apparent needs of specialties. It seems that a proportion of this perpetual motion (and loss) is due to one or other kind of stress avoidance or defensiveness, and again we should insist on asking why. And, revolutionary though the suggestion may be, we should question whether in our field competitiveness is an unqualified good.

There should be more insistence on having available whatever time the work takes – including whatever kind of supervision or personal or team consultation it takes to keep the work intelligently and thoughtfully on track and those involved in good shape. *This* is what is needed to make healthcare, 'care in the community' and other forms of care operate humanely and effectively – not endless inquiries, suspensions and the parrot cry 'lessons have been learned'. They never are, because the critical episodes are always different. This too is intrinsic to the field's complexity.

References

Anderson H (1995) Collaborative language systems: towards a postmodern therapy. In: R Mikesell, D Lusterman and S McDaniel (eds) *Integrating Family Therapy*. American Psychological Association, Washington, DC.

Anderson H (1997) *Conversation, Language and Possibilities: a postmodern approach to therapy*. Basic Books, New York.

Anderson H and Burney J (1999) Collaborative enquiry: a postmodern approach to organizational consultation. In: A Cooklin (ed) *Changing Organisations*. Karnac Books, London, pp 117–40.

Attenborough R (1985) *Arts and Disabled Report of Committee of Enquiry Under the Chairmanship of Richard Attenborough*. Carnegie Trust and Bedford Square Press, London.

Auerbach S (2001) Do patients want control over their own health care? *Journal of Health Psychology*. **6**: 191–203.

Balint M (1968) *The Doctor, His Patient and the Illness*. Pitman, London.

Bateson G (1973) *Steps to an Ecology of Mind*. Paladin Books, St Albans.

Bateson G (1979) *Mind and Nature: a necessary unity*. Wildwood House, London.

Bateson G, Jackson D, Haley J and Weakland J (1956) Towards a theory of schizophrenia. *Behavioural Science*. **1**: 251–65.

Baudrillard J (1983) *Simulations*. Semiotext, New York.

Beaver K, Luker K, Owens R, Leinster S, Degner L and Sloan J (1996) Treatment decision-making in women recently diagnosed with breast cancer. *Cancer Nursing*. **19**: 8–19.

Berger P and Luckman T (1997) *The Social Construction of Reality*. Penguin, Harmondsworth.

Blackmore S (1999) *The Meme Machine*. Oxford University Press, Oxford.

Bloch S and Harari E (2000) Family therapy. In: M Gelder, J Lopez-Ibor and N Andreasen (eds) *The New Oxford Textbook of Psychiatry*. Oxford University Press, Oxford, pp 1472–83.

Bloom H (2002) *Genius*. Fourth Estate, London.

Bowlby J (1949) *Child Care and the Growth of Love*. Penguin, Harmondsworth.

Bowlby J (1969) *Attachment and Loss. Vol 1: Attachment*. Hogarth Press, London.

Bowlby J (1973) *Attachment and Loss. Vol 2: Separation, anxiety and anger*. Hogarth Press, London.

Bowlby J (1980) *Attachment and Loss. Vol 3: Loss.* Hogarth Press, London.

Brown JAC (1961) *Freud and the Post-Freudians.* Penguin, Harmondsworth.

Brudenelle P (1987) Dramatherapy with people with a mental handicap. In: S Jennings (ed.) *Dramatherapy: theory and practice for teachers and clinicians.* Croom Helm, London.

Burton C (2002) Introduction to complexity. In: K Sweeney and F Griffiths (eds) *Complexity and Healthcare.* Radcliffe Medical Press, Oxford, pp 1–18.

Butler S (1922) *Erewhon.* Sage and Company, London.

Byrne A, Morton J and Salmon P (2001) Defending against patients' suffering: a qualitative analysis of children's post-operative pain. *Journal of Psychosomatic Research.* **50**: 69–76.

Campbell J (1974) *The Masks of God: Volume 4 – Creative Mythology.* Viking, London.

Campbell D (1999) Connecting personal experience to the primary task: a model for consulting to organisations. In: A Cooklin (ed.) *Changing Organisations.* Karnac Books, London, pp. 43–62.

Caplan C (1964) *Principles of Preventive Psychiatry.* Tavistock Publications, London.

Caplan C (1970) *The Principles and Practice of Mental Health Consultation.* Tavistock Publications, London.

Conoley JC and Conoley CW (1982) *School Consultation: a guide to practice and training.* Pergamon, New York.

Cooklin A (1999) *Changing Organisations: clinicians as agents of change.* Karnac Books, London and New York.

Coulter A (2003) Patients, power and responsibility. Review of Spiers (2003). *Journal of the Royal Society of Medicine.* **96**: 512–13.

Damasio A (1999) *The Feeling of What Happens.* William Heinemann, London.

de Haan E (2004) *The Consulting Process as Drama: learning from King Lear.* Karnac, London.

Dennett D (1991) *Consciousness Explained.* Allen Lane, London.

Eisenberg L (1975) The ethics of intervention: acting amidst ambiguity. *Journal of Child Psychology and Psychiatry.* **16**: 93–104.

Fitzpatrick M (2000) *The Tyranny of Health.* Brunner Routledge, London.

Furedi F (2004) *Therapy Culture: cultivating vulnerability in an uncertain age.* Routledge, London.

Foskett J (1986) The staff group. In: D Steinberg (ed.) *The Adolescent Unit: work and teamwork in adolescent psychiatry.* John Wiley, Chichester.

Foucault M (1967) *Madness and Civilization.* Tavistock, London.

Frank A (1997) *The Wounded Storyteller.* University of Chicago Press, Chicago, IL.

Gleick J (1987) *Chaos.* Penguin, Harmondsworth.

Gorell Barnes G (1994) Family therapy. In: M Rutter, E Taylor and L Hersor (eds) *Child and Adolescent Psychiatry: modern approaches*. Blackwell Scientific Publications, Oxford.

Guadagnoli E and Ward P (1998) Patient participation in decision-making. *Social Science and Medicine*. **47**: 329–39.

Higgs R (2003) The medical paradigm: changing landscapes. In: D Kirklin and R Richardson (eds) *The Healing Environment*. Royal College of Physicians, London.

Hinshelwood R (1994) *Clinical Klein*. Free Association Books, London.

Holmes J (1993) *John Bowlby and Attachment Theory*. Routledge, London.

Huyse F (1997) From consultation to complexity of care prediction and health service needs assessment (editorial). *Journal of Psychosomatic Research*. **43**: 233–40.

Huyse F (2000) The organisation of psychiatric services for general hospital departments. In: M Gelder, J Lopez-Ibor and N Andreasen (eds) *The New Oxford Textbook of Psychiatry*. Oxford University Press, Oxford, pp 1237–42.

Jennings S (ed.) (1987) *Dramatherapy: theory and practice for teachers and clinicians*. Croom Helm, London.

Jung CG (1964) *Man and His Symbols*. Aldus Books, London.

Kaye C (1997) State of the art. In: C Kaye and T Blee (eds) *The Arts in Health Care*. Jessica Kingsley Publishers, London.

Kernick D (2002) Complexity and healthcare organisation. In: K Sweeney and F Griffiths (eds) *Complexity and Healthcare: an introduction*. Radcliffe Medical Press, Oxford.

Kirklin D and Richardson R (eds) (2003) *The Healing Environment Without and Within*. Royal College of Physicians, London.

Kleinman A (1988) *The Illness Narratives*. Basic Books, New York.

Kubacki A (2003) *Journal of the Royal Society of Medicine*. **96**: 314 (correspondence).

Langer E (1989) *Mindfulness*. Addison-Wesley, Reading, MA.

Launer J (1996) 'You're the doctor, Doctor': is social constructionism a helpful stance in general practice consultations? *Journal of Family Therapy*. **18**: 255–67.

Launer J (2002) *Narrative-based Primary Care*. Radcliffe Medical Press, Oxford.

Like R and Zyzanski S (1987) Patient satisfaction with the clinical encounter: social psychological determinants. *Social Science and Medicine*. **24**(4): 351–7.

Lings P, Evans P, Seamark C, Sweeney K, Dixon M and Gray DP (2003) The doctor–patient relationship in US primary care. *Journal of the Royal Society of Medicine*. **96**: 180–4.

Lyotard J-F (1992) *The Postmodern Condition: a report on knowledge*. Manchester University Press, Manchester.

Mandelbrot B (1977) *The Fractal Geometry of Nature*. Freeman, New York.

McCleod J (1997) *Narrative and Psychotherapy*. Sage, London.

Menzies I (1970) *The Functioning of Social Systems as a Defence Against Anxiety*. Tavistock Pamphlet No. 3. Centre for Applied Social Research, Tavistock Institute of Human Relations, London.

Menzies Lyth I (1988) *Containing Anxiety in Institutions*. Free Association Books, London.

Miles M (1994) Art in hospitals: does it work? A survey of evaluation of arts projects in the NHS. *Proceedings of the Royal Society of Medicine*. **87**: 161–3.

Norris C (1987) *Derrida*. Fontana, London.

Ornstein R and Sobel D (1988) *The Healing Brain: a radical new approach to health care*. Macmillan, London.

Parry-Jones WL (1986) Multi-disciplinary teamwork: help or hindrance? In: D Steinberg (ed.) *The Adolescent Unit: work and teamwork in adolescent psychiatry*. John Wiley, Chichester.

Pattison S and Pill R (eds) (2004) *Values in Professional Practice*. Radcliffe Publishing, Oxford.

Pemberton M (2004) Trust Me – I'm a Junior Doctor. *The Daily Telegraph*. **July 30**.

Pendleton D, Schofield T, Tate P and Havelock P (2003) *The New Consultation: developing doctor-patient communication*. Oxford University Press, Oxford.

Peninsula Medical School (2005) *Undergraduate Prospectus: The Future of Healthcare*. Universities of Exeter and Plymouth.

Penrose R (1990) *The Emperor's New Mind*. Oxford University Press, Oxford.

Pichot P (2000) The history of psychiatry as a medical specialty. In: M Gelder, J Lopez-Ibor and N Andreasen (eds) *The New Oxford Textbook of Psychiatry*. Oxford University Press, Oxford.

Pinker S (1994) *The Language Instinct*. Penguin, London.

Pinker S (2002) *The Blank Slate*. Penguin, London.

Plsek P and Greenhalgh T (2001) The challenge of complexity in healthcare. *British Medical Journal*. **323**: 625–8.

Plsek P and Wilson T (2001) Complexity, leadership and management in healthcare organisations. *British Medical Journal*. **323**: 746–9.

Popper K (1999) *Unended Quest*. Routledge, London and New York.

Revans R (1962) The hospital as a human system. *Physics in Medicine and Biology*, reprinted (1990) in *Behavioural Science*. **35**, and quoted in Kaye 1997.

Rogers C (1951) *Client-centred Therapy*. Houghton-Mifflin, Boston, MA.

Salmon P and Hall G (2001) Patient-controlled analgesia or politically correct analgesia? *British Journal of Anaesthesia*. **87**: 815–18.

Salmon P and Hall G (2004) Patient empowerment or the emperor's new clothes? *Journal of the Royal Society of Medicine*. **97**: 53–6.

Schachar R and Ickowicz A (2000) Attention-deficit hyperkinetic disorders in childhood and adolescence. In: M Gelder, J Lopez-Ibor and N Andreasen (eds) *The New Oxford Textbook of Psychiatry*. Oxford University Press, Oxford.

Schlapobersky J (1989) *Institutes and How to Survive Them: Mental health training and consultation*. Selected papers by Robin Skynner. Methuen, London.

Silverstone L (1993) *Art Therapy the Person-Centred Way*. Autonomy Books, London.

Skynner R (1975) The large group in training. In: L Kreeger (ed.) *The Large Group: dynamics and therapy*. Constable, London.

Skynner R (1989) *Institutes and How to Survive Them: mental health training and consultation*. Essays, edited by J Schlapobersky. Routledge, London.

Sluzki C (1999) Language, practices and record-keeping: a reflective consultation and some institutional changes that resulted from it. In: A Cooklin (ed.) *Changing Organisations: clinicians as agents of change*. Karnac Books, London and New York, pp 27–42.

Spiers J (2003) *Patients, Power and Responsibility: the first principles of consumer-driven reform*. Radcliffe Medical Press, Oxford.

Staricoff R and Loppert S (2003) Integrating the arts into health care: can we affect clinical outcomes? In: D Kirklin and R Richardson (eds) *The Healing Environment*. Royal College of Physicians, London.

Steinberg D (1981) *Using Child Psychiatry: the functions and operations of a specialty*. Hodder and Stoughton, London.

Steinberg D (1982) Treatment, training, care or control? The functions of adolescent units. *British Journal of Psychiatry*. **141**: 306-9.

Steinberg D (1983) *The Clinical Psychiatry of Adolescence: clinical work from a social and developmental perspective*. John Wiley, Chichester.

Steinberg D (ed.) (1986a) *The Adolescent Unit: work and teamwork in adolescent psychiatry*. John Wiley, Chichester.

Steinberg D (1986b) Developments in a psychiatric service for adolescents. In: D Steinberg (ed.) *The Adolescent Unit: work and teamwork in adolescent psychiatry*. John Wiley, Chichester.

Steinberg D (1987) *Basic Adolescent Psychiatry*. Blackwell Science, Oxford.

Steinberg D (1989a) *Inter-Professional Consultation: innovation and imagination in working relationships*. Blackwell Science, Oxford.

Steinberg D, Wilson M and Acharyya S (1989b) 'My body hurts, my spirit hurts': the relationship between body, mind and soul. In: *Proceedings of a Conference on Assessment and Treatment Across Cultures*. Nafsyat: the Inter-Cultural Therapy Centre, London, pp 80–2.

Steinberg D (1991) Achievement in failure: working with staff in dangerous situations. Report of the International Conference on Children and Death, Athens, 1989. In: C Papadatos and D Papadatou (eds) *Children and Death*. Hemisphere Publishing, Washington, DC.

Steinberg D (1992) Informed consent: consultation as a basis for collaboration between disciplines and between professionals and their patients. *Journal of Interprofessional Care.* **61**: 43–8.

Steinberg D (1993a) Consultative work in child and adolescent psychiatry. In: M Garralda (ed.) *Managing Children with Psychiatric Problems.* BMJ Publishing Group, London.

Steinberg D (1993b) Psychiatry: concepts, principles and practicalities. In: C Brook (ed.) *The Practice of Medicine in Adolescence.* Edward Arnold, London, pp 35–44.

Steinberg D (2000a) The child psychiatrist as consultant to schools and colleges. In: M Gelder, J Lopez-Ibor and N Andreasen (eds) *The New Oxford Textbook of Psychiatry.* Oxford University Press, Oxford.

Steinberg D (2000b) *Letters From the Clinic: letter writing in clinical practice for mental health professionals.* Brunner Routledge, London.

Steinberg D (2000c) *The Future of Adolescent Psychiatry.* Report of a lecture given at the National Congress on Adolescent Psychiatry, Okayama, 2000. UNI Agency Inc., Tokyo.

Steinberg D (2000d) Inter-professional consultation and creative approaches in therapeutic work across cultures. In: J Kareem and R Littlewood (eds) *Inter-cultural Therapy* (2e). Blackwell Science, Oxford.

Steinberg D (2004a) From archetype to impressions: the magic of words. In: G Bolton, S Howlett, C Lago and J Wright (eds) *Writing Cures.* Brunner Routledge, London.

Steinberg D (2004b) Child and adolescent psychiatry – a model for medical teaching. *Journal of the Royal Society of Medicine.* **97**: 545–6.

Steinberg D (forthcoming) *Consciousness Reconnected: missing links between neuroscience, depth psychology and the arts.* Radcliffe Publishing, Oxford.

Steinberg D, Galhenage D and Robinson S (1981) Two years' referrals to a regional adolescent unit: some implications for psychiatric services. *Social Science and Medicine.* **15**: 113–22.

Steinberg D and Hughes L (1987) The emergence of work-centred issues in consultative work: an observation. *Journal of Adolescence.* **10**: 309–16.

Stevens A (1982) *Archetype: a natural history of the self.* Routledge and Kegan Paul, London.

Stevens A (1990) *On Jung.* Penguin Books, London.

Storr A (1998) *The Essential Jung.* Fontana, London.

Sukkar M, El-Munshid H and Ardawi M (2000) *Concise Human Physiology* (2e). Blackwell Science, Oxford.

Sulloway F (1979) *Freud: biologist of the mind.* Andre Deutsch, London.

Sweeney K and Griffiths F (2002) *Complexity and Healthcare: an introduction.* Radcliffe Medical Press, Oxford.

Tattum D (1986) *The Management of Disruptive Behaviour in Schools.* John Wiley, Chichester.

Topping K (1986) Consultative enhancement of school-based action. In: D

Tattum (1986) *The Management of Disruptive Behaviour in Schools*. John Wiley, Chichester.

Tyrer P and Steinberg D (2005) *Models for Mental Disorder* (4e). John Wiley, London and Chichester.

Ulrich R (1984) View through a window may influence recovery from surgery. *Science*. 420–1.

Ulrich R (1992) How design impacts wellness. *Healthcare Forum Journal*. **10**: 20–5.

Vitebsky P (1995) *The Shaman*. Duncan Baird Publishers, London.

Von Bertalanffy L (1968) *General Systems Theory*. George Brazillier, New York.

Wall A (2003) Mind your language. *Journal of the Royal Society of Medicine*. **96**: 357–8.

Waterworth S and Luker K (1990) Reluctant collaborators: do patients want to be involved in decisions concerning care? *Journal of Advanced Nursing*. **15**: 971–6.

Wilkinson J (2000) *Music in Healthcare Project: evaluation report*. Music Network 2000, Dublin.

Winnicott D (1972) *The Maturational Process and the Facilitating Environment*. Hogarth Press, London.

Winnicott D (1988) *Human Nature*. Free Association Books, London.

Wollheim R (1971) *Freud*. Fontana Modern Masters series. Fontana/Collins, London.

Index